TRIAL BY FURY

TRIAL
BY DISCARDED
FURY

THE POLIO VACCINE CONTROVERSY

Aaron E. Klein

Charles Scribner's Sons
New York

To
Samuel Klein,
Robert Themper,
George Lee—
all my fathers

CONTENTS

A Selection of Pictures   xi
I. The Wages of Virtue   3
II. Public Relations and Polio   10
III. The Influenza Apprenticeship   24
IV. The End of Orthodoxy   42
V. A Hero Is Created   66
VI. A Time for Impatience   86
VII. The Sting of the Needle   102
VIII. Syrup and Sugar Cubes   127
Epilogue   152

Glossary   161
Chronology   164
Bibliography   166
Index   169

A
SELECTION
OF
PICTURES

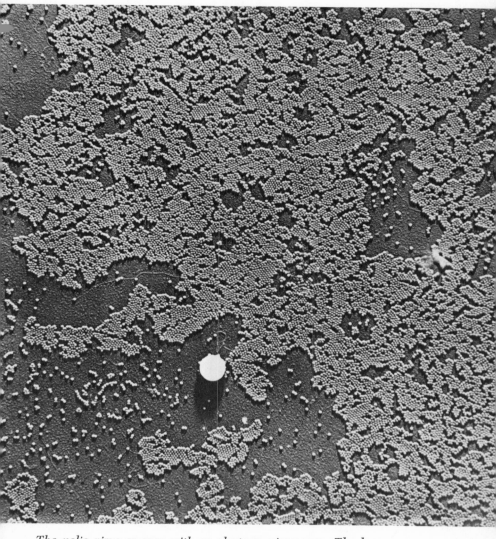

The polio virus as seen with an electron microscope. The large white spot is a sphere of known size placed in the preparation as a measuring device

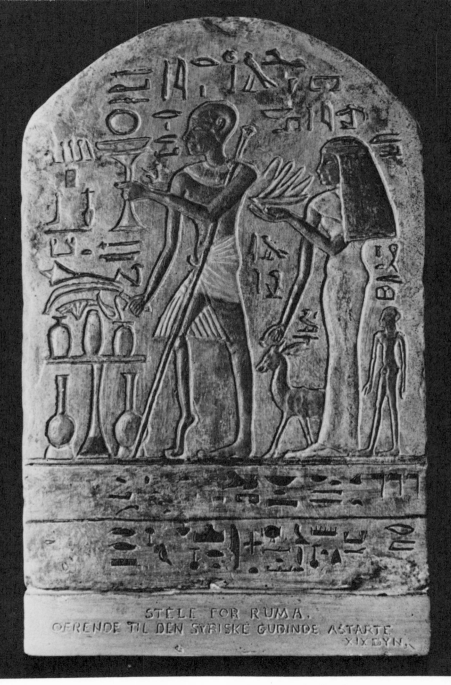

An Egyptian stele showing possible polio victim

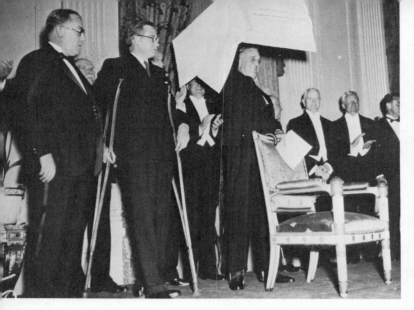

(Above) President Franklin D. Roosevelt displaying a giant replica of a check for $1,003,030.08—the proceeds from the 1934 series of President's Birthday Balls; at far left, Basil O'Connor

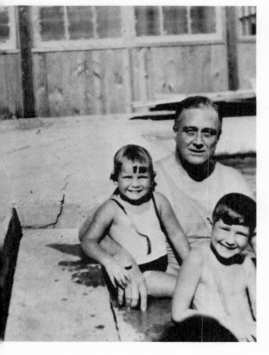

Roosevelt and two young patients at Warm Springs, Georgia

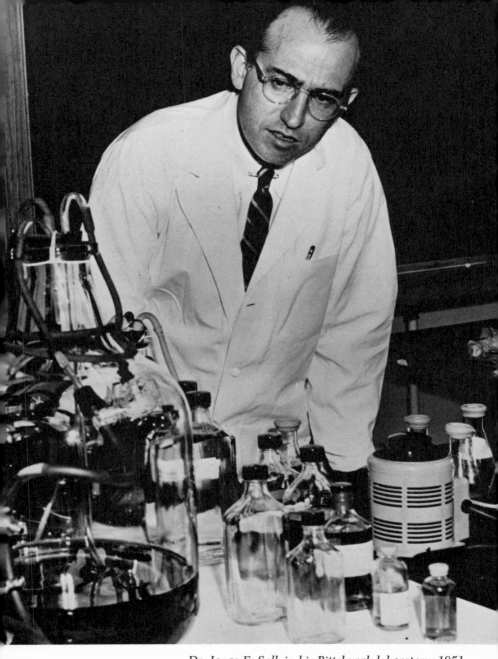

Dr. Jonas E. Salk in his Pittsburgh laboratory, 1951

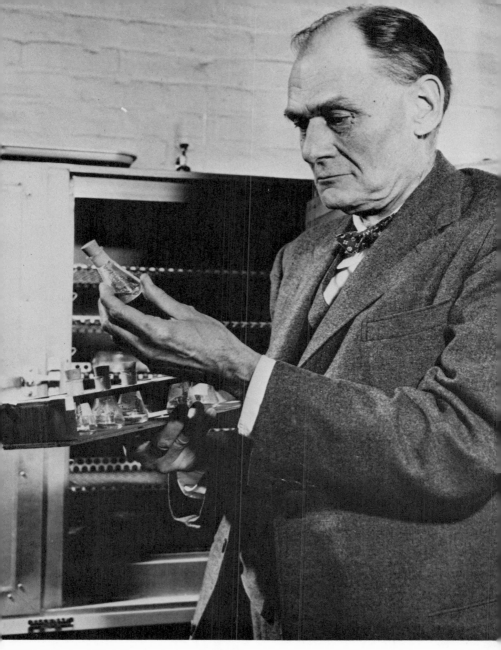

Dr. John F. Enders in his Boston laboratory

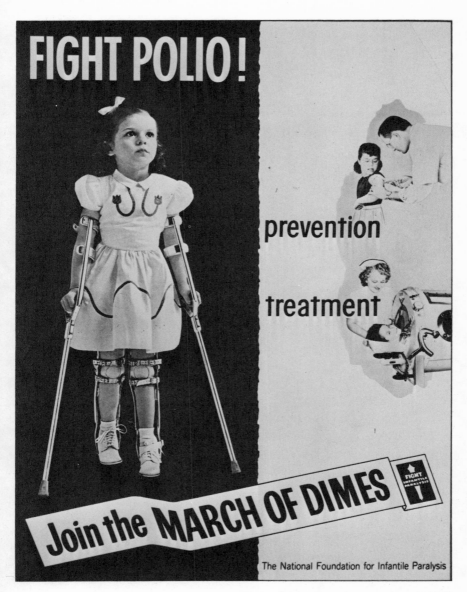

Typical March of Dimes poster (1955)

Rounding Third!

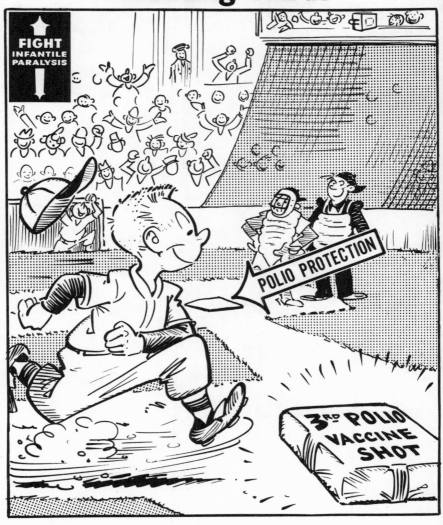

Promotion poster for the vaccination campaign (1957)

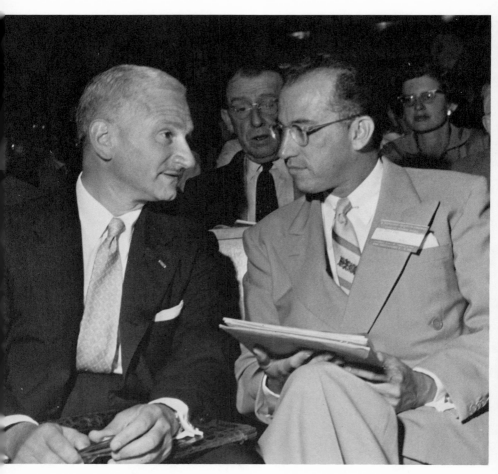

Dr. Albert B. Sabin and Dr. Salk at the Third International Poliomyelitis Congress in Rome, 1953; behind them is Basil O'Connor

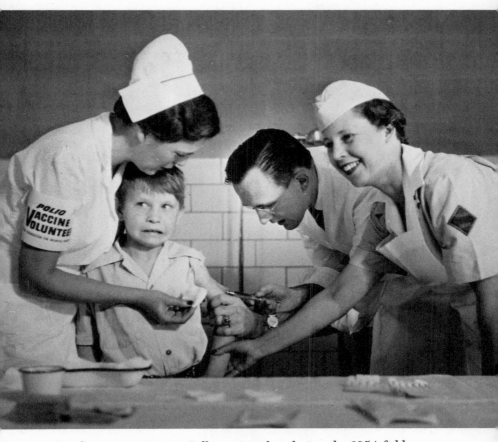

A volunteer receiving a Salk vaccine shot during the 1954 field trials

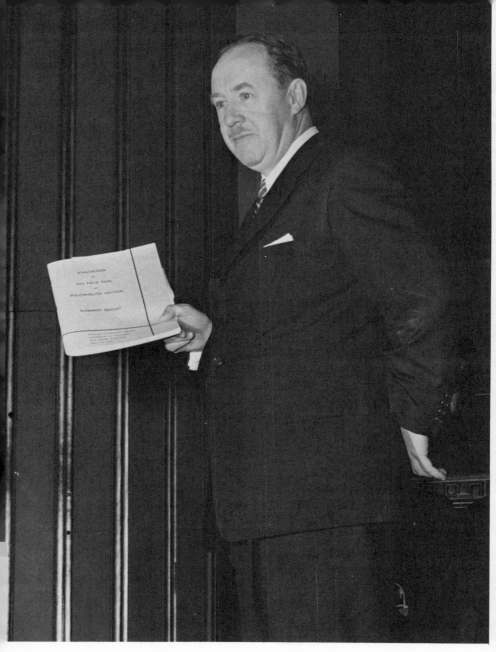

Dr. Thomas Francis with the evaluation report of the Salk vaccine field trials, Ann Arbor, Michigan, April 12, 1955

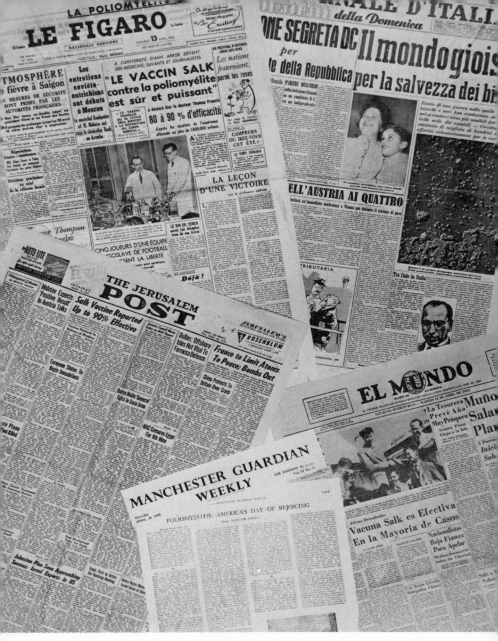

Some reactions of the world press to the evaluation report

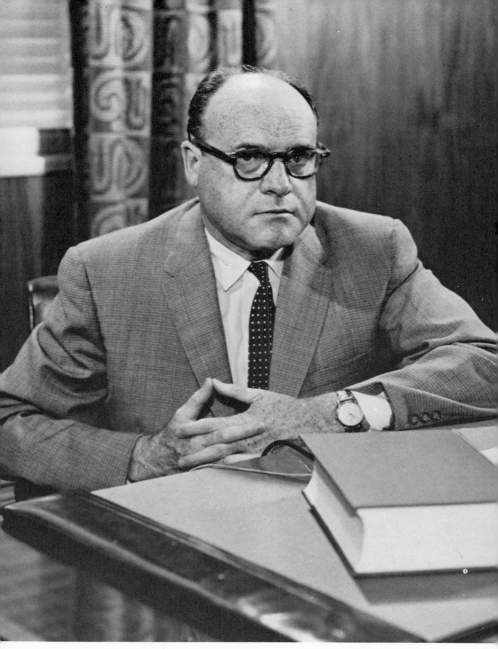

Dr. Herald Cox

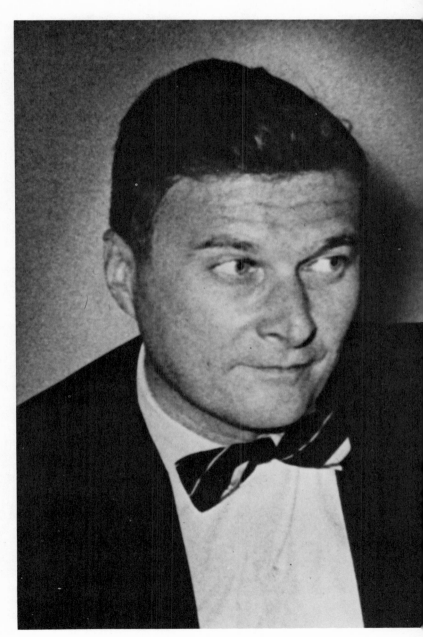

Dr. Hilary Koprowski

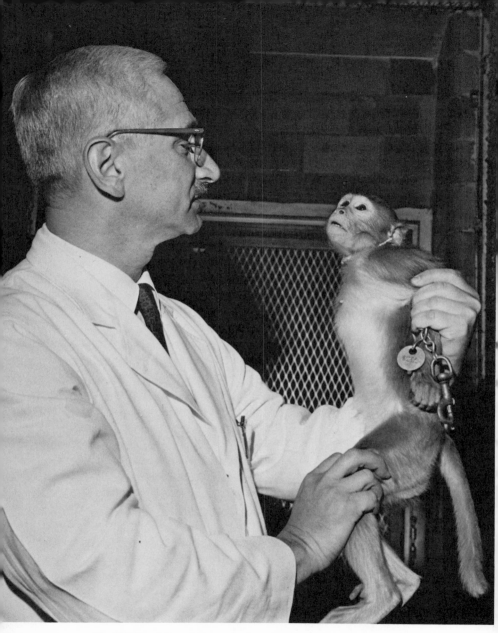

Dr. Sabin with a rhesus monkey

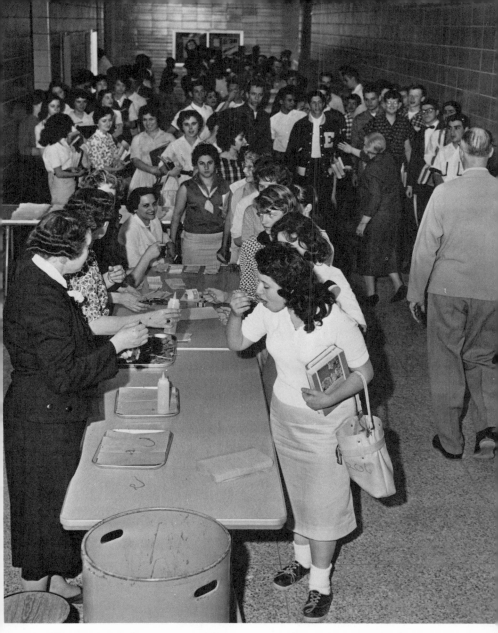

Dispensing Sabin vaccine in a syrup medium to high-school students during the 1960 oral vaccine campaign

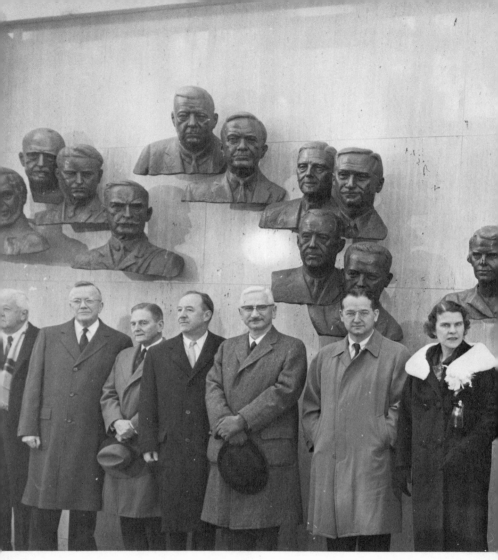

At the dedication of the Polio Hall of Fame at Warm Springs in January 1958. The frieze in the background shows the busts of the seventeen persons named to the Hall of Fame. The recipients of the honor who were present are (left to right): Dr. Thomas M. Rivers, Dr. Charles Armstrong, Dr. John R. Paul, Dr. Thomas Francis, Dr. Albert B. Sabin, Dr. Joseph L. Melnick, Dr. Isabel Morgan, Dr. Howard A. Howe, Dr. David Bardian, Dr. Jonas E. Salk, Mrs. Franklin D. Roosevelt (representing her husband), Basil O'Connor

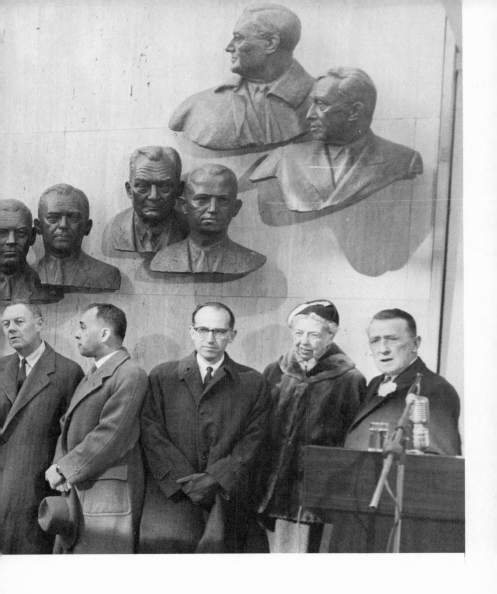

TRIAL BY FURY

THE
WAGES
OF
VIRTUE

Most of the great epidemic diseases of man, such as the Black Plague, are associated with centuries past. Not so poliomyelitis. That one belongs to us.

Although this disease has been around a long time —there is evidence, obtained from the bones of a mummy, that an Egyptian pharaoh may have had it— poliomyelitis did not occur in large epidemics or attract a great deal of attention until the present century. In the industrialized countries of the world with a high standard of living, such as the United States, Great Britain, and Sweden, poliomyelitis in the first half of this century struck like a plague. Since it was a disease of children, so much so that it was generally called infantile paralysis, outbreaks were accompanied by a

3

great deal of emotional terror. The terror was not the mass hysteria which characterized the Black Plague of the fourteenth century but a quiet dread in the minds of parents, who lived with the fear that at any time the virus of poliomyelitis could paralyze or kill their children.

There was nothing doctors could do for the victims other than massage limbs, put paralyzed legs in steel braces, and place those with paralyzed muscles of breathing in iron lungs. When the disease became a major problem, medical scientists started programs of research. Scientists had found ways to control other diseases, and it seemed likely that poliomyelitis could be dispatched as readily as diphtheria and typhoid fever had been in the late nineteenth and early twentieth centuries. But poliomyelitis, the twentieth-century affliction, defied all efforts of early twentieth-century scientists to find a cure or prevention. No one realized at the time that the successful efforts of nineteenth-century bacteriologists and other scientists to bring a host of other infectious diseases under control had paved the way for the spectacular debut of poliomyelitis epidemics in the twentieth century.

There were a few minor outbreaks of poliomyelitis in the late nineteenth century, but these scattered cases attracted little attention from either the general public or medical men. During these same and preceding years, children had died by the thousands from such diseases as diphtheria, typhoid, and tuberculosis. Poliomyelitis was a relatively rare disease that seldom caused death, and medical researchers just did not have time for it. They found a lot of time for diphtheria and typhoid, and in the first two decades of this century these diseases were slowly being brought under control.

The discovery of the bacterial causes of various infectious diseases and the consequent development of cures and vaccines certainly helped. Just as important in the eventual eradication of these diseases was the realization that disease organisms could be carried in media such as milk and contaminated water supplies. Many cities and states then required the pasteurization of milk and improved their water and sewage systems.

The association of disease-causing organisms with dirt and filth led to a new popularity for cleanliness. Daily bathing, which had long been considered to be an unhealthy practice, was vigorously promoted. Hospitals, cleaner than they ever were before, smelled of strong antiseptics. Doctors who washed their hands and steamed their instruments before operations were no longer laughed out of the profession.

Through articles in newspapers, magazines, and Sunday supplements, people in advanced countries such as the United States became very much aware of the invisible multitude of disease organisms conveniently called "germs." Many school districts required that their children receive instruction in "health and hygiene," and Congress passed laws intended to protect the citizenry from dirty food and phony medicines.

Babies especially came to be fiercely protected, and campaigns were undertaken to introduce mothers to the new regime of cleanliness. Everything intended to come into contact with the inside or outside of baby was boiled, steamed, or disinfected to kill the evil "germs." Visiting nurses, some on the backs of mules, carried the sanitary doctrine to isolated corners of the country. As hospital hygiene improved, more and more women gave birth to babies in hospitals, attended by doctors, rather than at home under the frequently dubious care of "unsanitary" midwives.

By the second decade of the twentieth century Americans could proudly point to statistics that showed that many fewer babies died in their first year than had been the case before. The statistics were particularly impressive if one ignored the figures from the non-white population of the rural South, where conditions were as bad as they had ever been. Elsewhere the death rates from infectious diseases slowly dropped, and insurance companies were particularly pleased as the average life expectancy increased. Many Americans felt smugly superior to the poor unfortunates in less enlightened countries who knew nothing of simple hygiene. And poliomyelitis was only an interesting word one might find in a medical dictionary.

Poliomyelitis quite suddenly became much more than just an interesting word when, in 1916, a massive epidemic broke out in the United States. Before it was over there were some 27,000 cases and over 6000 deaths. In some parts of the country, especially New York, the people reacted as though a plague had struck. In panic thousands attempted to flee the city, and in some localities the New Yorkers were turned away by armed citizens who were afraid that the city people would bring the infection into their towns.

Earlier epidemics of such diseases as yellow fever and cholera had had much higher case totals and death tolls, and the influenza pandemic that would follow in two years would eclipse the 1916 poliomyelitis epidemic in terms of numbers of people affected; but even though the number of poliomyelitis cases and deaths was relatively small, its effects and its apparent propensity for children made this disease particularly terrible. When other epidemics had run their course the survivors recuperated and the dead were buried and forgotten. The victims of poliomyelitis could not be so easily forgotten, for many of the survivors were permanently paralyzed.

To many Americans the outbreak of poliomyelitis was an affront to national pride. Everybody had been taught that cleanliness prevented disease, and people were shocked that such a disaster could happen in their hygienic country. This epidemic was the kind of thing that was supposed to happen in primitive countries with no sewers or waterworks, not in the clean, modern United States of 1916. Why had this disease waited until the twentieth century to break out in epidemic proportions? Why did outbreaks seem to occur mainly in "enlightened" countries such as the United States and Sweden? No one knew it at the time, but the reason was the mania for cleanliness and the desire to protect children from "germs."

Children are naturally exposed to disease organisms from the moment of birth. They may come down with a variety of diseases from which they either recover or die. Recovery from a disease usually results in immunity to that particular disease—that is, the body builds up a resistance to the specific disease-causing organism. In the case of many diseases, it is not necessary to become noticeably sick to develop an immunity. Poliomyelitis is one of these.

Poliomyelitis is ordinarily a mild, viral infection of the intestinal tract. Most babies are born with a temporary, partial, or complete immunity to many diseases, including poliomyelitis. If a baby is exposed to the virus of poliomyelitis while it has the temporary immunity, it will develop a stronger, more permanent immunity; its mild discomfort will be unnoticed in the process. If the baby has no contact with this virus, the temporary immunity of infancy will wear away. Most American babies, carefully guarded from every speck of dirt and dust, have little opportunity to develop a natural immunity to poliomyelitis or anything else. Under these sheltered conditions great havoc can be caused if the poliomyelitis virus particles break out of the intestines into the bloodstream and are carried to all parts of the body. It is when the virus enters nerve cells in the brain and spinal cord and destroys or damages these cells that the paralytic symptoms of poliomyelitis become evident.

The name "poliomyelitis" is somewhat of a misnomer. It means "inflammation of the gray matter of the spinal cord," from the Greek *polio*, which means "gray," and *myel*, which refers to the spinal cord. As the disease increased in incidence and became familiar to everyone, it was called simply "polio." Most people did not know they were calling a disease "gray," and no one knew that tens of thousands of people had already had the disease without being aware of it.

When the relationship between clean living and polio came to be understood, no one proposed giving dirty milk to babies or feeding them from unwashed dishes just so they might develop an immunity to polio. Other diseases had been controlled by injecting immunity-causing substances into willing or unwilling recipients, and to develop the same sort of thing for polio seemed to be the thing to do.

Some forty years were to go by after the first polio epidemic of 1916 before a way was found to immunize people against polio. The research campaign against polio was to be the largest voluntarily funded program of research ever directed at a specific infectious disease. In the 1930s an organization, the National Foundation for Infantile Paralysis, was established for the sole purpose of collecting contributions and doling the money out to scientists. People were now in a desperate hurry for the polio terror to end, and great demands were made on the scientists to produce quickly. The pressure from the foundation and the contributing public frequently forced a relaxation of the necessarily meticulous, carefully controlled, and consequently slow methods of the laboratory scientist, and the result was repeated tragedy before the goal of a safe polio vaccine was finally attained.

PUBLIC
RELATIONS
AND
POLIO

CHAPTER II

IMMEDIATELY FOLLOWING THE 1916 epidemic there was no great movement to start a research program to find a cure or prevention for polio. Although cases continued to occur, there were no more great epidemics until the late 1920s. When the severity of epidemics increased in the 1930s and 1940s, polio attracted more attention, and the demand for research increased.

Those who wanted to sponsor a research campaign against polio discovered a few hard, bitter facts. Scientific research was very expensive. If a large research program was to be carried out, large amounts of money had to be gathered. In the United States of the 1930s the sources of money for scientific work were limited to individual philanthropies, a few endowed universities and foundations, and a few generous corporations.

The chaotic condition of science-funding goes back to the origins of experimental science.

Science as we know it today began to develop during the eighteenth century in a period that has been called the "Age of Enlightenment." Early scientists were called "gentlemen scientists"—for good reason. Although early scientific efforts were not very expensive, they did require a great deal of time. A scientist therefore had to be in a position where he did not have to work for a living. Most of the early scientists were wealthy and titled gentlemen who had the means, and therefore the time, to devote to scientific activities. In some eras, kings, princes, and other men of means became "patrons" of science by providing money for scientists.

By the late nineteenth century some governments were assuming a role in science-funding (Louis Pasteur was in the employ of the French government when he did some of his most significant work). But scientists directly in the employ of government were and still are in the minority. This has been the case especially in the United States, with its tradition of free enterprise. Generally most scientists became associated with universities. The universities provided gainful employment and a place to carry out research, but they could not always provide the necessary money for the research itself. Much of this money came from outside sources—ranging from governments to eccentric millionaires. The obtaining of grants of money came to be a mark of prestige for scientists and for the universities that housed them.

One of the unfortunate aspects of grants is that they frequently come from groups that want fast, specific answers to practical problems, whether it is the development of a more powerful bomb or the cure for a disease. What is frequently overlooked by the generous suppliers of money is that scientists are not magicians or miracle workers. Usually basic scientific information is needed before practical solutions to practical problems can be obtained. While most scientists prefer to do basic research, donors are usually reluctant to provide money for basic research that does not seem immediately relevant to what they want. Industrialists who employ scientists at great expense and foundations dedicated to the conquest of specific diseases have discovered that much basic research is needed before their goals can be reached.

The success of the bacteriologists in the late nineteenth and early twentieth centuries stimulated the formation of many foundations aimed at controlling diseases. Many of these, such as the American Cancer Society and the American Heart Association, originated as organizations of doctors. Others were started by interested laymen. One of the first laymen's groups was a "modest" society organized in Philadelphia in 1890, to provide information about a "cure" for tuberculosis. This group eventually became the National Tuberculosis Association.

The activities of the National Tuberculosis Association certainly contributed to the spectacular dip in

the tuberculosis death rate, though they have yet to result in a specific cure for tuberculosis. However, its or-
ganizers made a very significant discovery, which
eventually led to the conquest of many other diseases.
This discovery was that while philanthropists may always be in short supply, ordinary people can be per-
suaded to give small sums of money for a specific cause
if they can be convinced that the cause is worthy.

People are not usually eager to part with their
money unless they receive something tangible in return. The fund-raisers for the National Tuberculosis
Association soon found that if there was enough emotional appeal to the request for funds, people would
give. The emotional appeal in this case was the disease
itself. Tuberculosis was the leading killer of people in
the late nineteenth and early twentieth centuries. Perhaps many people unconsciously thought that their
small contributions were somewhat like the blood of
the lamb on the doorpost that would keep the plague
away from their homes. The appeal was tied up in a
neat little package with the first sale of Christmas seals
in 1907. Now there was even a tangible return for the
offering. The would-be polio conquerers were destined
to have the most powerful emotional appeal in the history of fund-raising.

Franklin D. Roosevelt was a promising young poli-
tician in 1920. Member of a prominent old American
family, relative of an ex-President, good-looking, solid
family man as he appeared to be, he had all the qualifications for high office. The Democrats had great hopes
when they nominated him to run for vice-president in
1920. The Democrats lost that election, but the figure

of Franklin D. Roosevelt still stood out as a possible future winner for the Democrats.

Following the election, Roosevelt and his family went to Campobello Island for a vacation. One morning, following a strenuous day of swimming and boating, he awoke with a fever. His illness was diagnosed as a severe case of polio. It resulted in the paralysis of his legs. This event was reported in newspapers all over the country and served to focus attention on a disease that had almost been forgotten by the general public in the years following the 1916 epidemic.

Roosevelt's fight against the disease was inspiring. He was a man of considerable means, and he could have retired to his home in Hyde Park, New York, and lived a pleasant life as a country gentleman. Instead he chose to overcome the disease as much as possible and to re-enter the field of politics. When he lifted himself up on his paralyzed legs to make the nominating speech for Alfred E. Smith at the Democratic National Convention of 1924, the dramatic effect was felt not only by the convention delegates but by the entire nation.

That year Roosevelt and Basil O'Connor, a Wall Street lawyer, formed a partnership. Both men saw great advantages in this. O'Connor had connections that could aid Roosevelt's political ambitions. Roosevelt, as a well-known political personality, could further O'Connor's law career.

During the 1920s Roosevelt spent a lot of time at a shabby resort hotel in the town of Warm Springs, Georgia. He thought that swimming in the naturally heated, buoyant waters might be beneficial. With some of his associates, he eventually bought the hotel, hoping to turn it into a health resort. After his election as Governor of New York in 1928, Roosevelt asked O'Connor to take over the administration of the resort. O'Connor agreed to do this, with great reluctance.

The resort was a financial disaster. Most of the crippled people who came there (largely polio victims) had no money, and non-crippled people with money preferred to spend their vacations at places where they would not have to look at cripples. The stock-market crash of 1929 cut off most sources of philanthropy. By the time Roosevelt was elected President of the United States in 1932, the resort had more unpaid bills than it had paying guests.

In the four years that O'Connor ran the place he developed an attachment for it and became determined to save it. He was convinced that the only way to do it was to solicit contributions from the public. The National Tuberculosis Association had shown that this could be done. O'Connor and Roosevelt consulted public-relations firms. American advertising and public-relations firms had been very successful in convincing people that one kind of toothpaste or cigarette was better than another, and Roosevelt and O'Connor felt that these companies could certainly think of ways to convince large numbers of people to give away a little of their money for a deserving cause.

After much thought the fund-raising campaign was tied to Roosevelt by making it a celebration of his birthday. Here was a perfect emotional symbol about which to build a campaign. The public-relations firms suggested that a series of "President's Birthday Balls" be organized. Money collected for admission tickets would be used to save the Warm Springs health resort.

Rallying to the slogan "To dance so that others may walk," the well-organized machinery of the Democratic party was utilized to plan balls in cities all over the country. This was in 1934, one of the worst years of the economic depression. Nevertheless the balls were successful, and over a million dollars was raised.

The 1935 and 1936 series of balls were disappointing. It was ironic that the very symbol O'Connor's group hoped to use to great advantage turned out to be somewhat of a liability. Roosevelt had by this time been president long enough to earn enemies and criticism. The Birthday Balls were too closely associated with Roosevelt and the Democratic party, and it was obvious that a new approach was needed.

After many conferences with O'Connor and more public-relations firms, Roosevelt announced that a foundation would be formed that would, among other things, "ensure that every responsible research agency in this country is adequately financed to carry out investigations into the cause of infantile paralysis and the methods by which it may be prevented" (*The New York Times*, September 23, 1937). The organization was called the National Foundation for Infantile Paralysis. Its president was, of course, Basil O'Connor, who immediately had to get down to the business of raising money. The year was 1938. The country had only partially recovered from the great depression. Philanthropists were still very hard to find, and the major fundraising thrust had to be appeals directly to the people for small contributions. A new slogan had to be devised, and advertising agencies were again consulted.

The slogan came, not from New York's advertising agencies, but from the make-believe capital of the world, Hollywood. Eddie Cantor, a popular radio and film comedian, suggested the slogan "The March of Dimes." This was apparently an allusion to a widely viewed, quasi-intellectual film documentary called *The March of Time*. In those days before television, *The March of Time* was shown as a short subject in movie theaters all over the country. It made viewers feel well informed on important events and trends of the day.

Cantor further suggested that radio stations be asked to donate short spots of time to broadcast appeals for people to send their dimes directly to President Roosevelt in the White House. The White House was certainly an easy address to remember, and the prospect of sending a dime to the president was sure to be fascinating to many people.

The appeals on radio, in newspapers, magazines, and other communications media reached a peak on January 30, 1938, the president's birthday. Two days later, exactly $17.50 had been received at the White House. It appeared that the March of Dimes had been the most colossal failure in the history of fund-raising. On the third day following the birthday the situation changed dramatically. So many bags of mail were delivered to the White House that there was no place to store them. The corridors of the White House were impassable. The official White House mail, communications from heads of state of other countries and other important letters, could not be found in the mess. Dimes had been sent baked in cakes, enclosed in gift-wrapped boxes, and wrapped in yards of tape. Along with money of other denominations, there were over 2,-600,000 dimes. Almost $2,000,000 was collected. The problem of how to raise money was apparently solved. Now a bigger problem faced the foundation—what to do with all this money. To this problem the sincere men of the foundation applied their full but cautious attention. The caution was the result of a disaster dating back to the Birthday Ball days.

Scientists have been criticized for being a secretive, aloof group who want to have as little contact as possible with the public. There is a reason for this apparent lack of communication between scientist and non-scientist. The esteem and respect of other scientists are very important to a person engaged in scientific work. Once a scientist has lost the respect of his colleagues it is difficult to find a good position, get one's research papers published, or receive grants. One of the quickest ways for a scientist to fall into disfavor is to make claims he cannot support with evidence.

Many scientists have fallen into disfavor with their colleagues as the result of newspaper accounts of their work. Reporters are known to exaggerate information related to them by scientists, as well as by politicians and other notables. A badly written newspaper story can make it appear that a scientist is making unfounded claims even if this is not really the case. Scientists are therefore reluctant to talk about their work, especially to reporters and other non-scientists who may misinterpret what they say.

When a scientist thinks he has something worth talking about, he will write a paper on his work and

submit it for publication in a scientific journal. This is
the safe, accepted way of passing on information
within the scientific fraternity. Journals are read only
by other scientists, usually only by those in the same
field of study as the writer. Most of the general public
does not even know the journals exist. The scientist is
protected from unwanted publicity. His colleagues
may disagree with him, but that is the way of science.
Even if he makes a mistake now and then, he is likely
to keep the respect of his colleagues.

Mass publicity, so deadly to a scientist, was vital
to an organization such as the foundation. Here lay the
seeds of trouble. The foundation had a lot of money to
dole out in grants to polio researchers. Scientists whose
fields of research impinged even slightly on the polio
problem were anxious to get some of this money. The
foundation felt that it had an obligation to let the contributors know what was being done with their money.
The scientists felt that they had an obligation to keep
silent until they were reasonably sure they had enough
professional evidence to say something. Many a polio
researcher later became annoyed with the foundation
people for making over-optimistic statements to the
press that were embarrassing to him.

Basil O'Connor and the Birthday Ball Commission
who had begun it all in 1935 were not scientists and
they knew it. They had appointed an American bacteriologist, Paul de Kruif, to look for scientists who might
be able to do useful things with the Birthday Ball
money. De Kruif had become fairly well known to the
general public after he left the laboratory to write popular books on science (the best known of which is the

classic *Microbe Hunters*). He started to look for somebody who could develop a polio vaccine. He should have known better.

Trying to develop a polio vaccine in 1935 was somewhat like a Stone Age man trying to invent an automobile. Next to nothing was known about the polio virus, or any other virus for that matter. Much of the little that was thought to be known was later shown to be misleading.

Nevertheless, Maurice Brodie, a young research worker at the New York University School of Medicine, said that he could make a polio vaccine. To that end, de Kruif saw to it that Brodie got $65,000. De Kruif had previously criticized O'Connor for putting all the money into Warm Springs, maintaining that no one had ever been cured of polio there.

Brodie injected polio virus into monkeys. He then ground up the spinal cords of the monkeys and put the ground-up material into formalin, a solution of formaldehyde gas in water. The formalin was supposed to kill the virus, assumed to be in the spinal cords. Brodie claimed that the killed-virus suspension could induce immunity to polio without causing the disease. He injected monkeys with the material, and in a dramatic gesture even injected himself. He claimed that when live polio virus was injected into the inoculated monkeys, they did not come down with polio. He therefore assumed that they were immune. Since Brodie continued to live after receiving the material, it was thought to be safe.

Brodie's vaccine was injected into hundreds of children. Brodie was hailed as the new Pasteur. The

Birthday Ball people were ecstatic. Then the adulation suddenly stopped. When other workers, repeating Brodie's experiments, injected live polio virus into monkeys "immunized" with Brodie's vaccine, the monkeys promptly died of polio. It was revealed that at least one child had died and three had come down with paralytic polio after receiving the vaccine.

This sad affair contributed to the disappointing results of the 1936 Birthday Balls. The cause was not helped by another disaster, which had nothing to do with the Birthday Ball Commission. A Dr. John Kolmer at Temple University in Philadelphia claimed to have developed a vaccine made from live viruses. Kolmer said that the viruses had been changed so that they would induce immunity but not produce symptoms of the disease. Of the thousands of children injected with this vaccine, six died and three were paralyzed. Apparently none of the children developed any immunity.

The publicity-conscious O'Connor group had been badly hurt by the publicity it had so eagerly sought. The expensive lesson learned was that much basic research was needed before anyone could try to make a vaccine, if indeed a vaccine was possible. Now, in 1939, the foundation acted more wisely. A Virus Research Committee was formed and a virologist, Dr. Thomas M. Rivers, was named to head this committee, which was responsible for reviewing requests for grants.

Rivers had been associated with the Birthday Ball Commission and had been director of the Rockefeller Hospital since 1929. Through his work at the Rockefeller Institute (now The Rockefeller University) and as author of several books on virology, he had established himself as one of the leading virologists in the country. He came from a small town in Georgia and looked and talked more like a redneck cotton farmer than a virologist. His term with the foundation was long and stormy, and at times he wielded more power in the organization than O'Connor himself. In matters of research, if Rivers was not in favor of it, the research was not likely to be approved. His brusque and often profane manner of putting down those who disagreed with him earned him many enemies, and he was always at the center of the foundation's controversies and crises until his death in 1962.

From 1938 on through World War II, the foundation did very well in fund-raising campaigns. The National Foundation for Infantile Paralysis was the best-publicized organization of its kind. Many people thought that it was a governmental agency and that the president's birthday was a national holiday. The men of the foundation had learned that no fast miracles were forthcoming, but they still relied heavily on massive publicity to keep going. The publicity would backfire in other disasters.

During the tragic years of the Brodie and Kolmer fiascos, a young man named Jonas Salk was quietly going about the business of getting his medical degree at New York University, the same institution at which Brodie worked on his vaccine. Another graduate of New York University Medical School, Albert Sabin, had just accepted a position at the Rockefeller Institute. Even at this early date Sabin was well along in making his place in virology, and he joined in the general outcry against Brodie and Kolmer. Salk was still a medical student, and if he was concerned with these events he told no one about it. The two men had no way of knowing at the time that they too would be caught in the wild, furious triumphs and tragedies of the foundation and its fight against polio.

THE
INFLUENZA
APPRENTICESHIP

CHAPTER III ▪▪▪▪▪▪▪▪▪▪▪▪▪▪▪▪▪▪

THAT JONAS SALK ENTERED THE
City College of New York at the age of fifteen surprised no one who knew him. His parents, for example,
expected nothing less, and they probably expected
a great deal more of their obviously very bright son.
The mid-adolescent college entry was according to
plan. Jonas was twelve when he started at Townsend
Harris High School, a rigorous, accelerated school run
by City College for exceptional boys. Young Salk consistently came out on top of the academic heap. Anything less was unthinkable.

For thousands of bright New York boys whose
parents were not financially well off, school was an
arena of combat in which all others were deadly competitors. It was not the violent combat of street gangs,

24

fought with fists, knives, and zip guns. It was a silent but intense combat, and the weapons were books, attentiveness at lectures, and examinations. The winners were those with the spongelike brains that could soak up the wisdom of the books and teachers the fastest, and squeeze it all out again in neat lines in examination booklets. The prize was escape.

One had to go college to get the diploma that was hopefully the ticket of escape from the tenements of the Lower East Side, Bronx, and Brooklyn. For Jonas Salk and thousands of other strivers, scholarships and free colleges were the only way to the degrees that were synonymous with "being somebody." Every point on an examination was bitterly contested, for that point might mean that someone else would have an average one-tenth of a point higher than yours and so get the scholarship that you needed.

Jonas Salk soaked up the course work at college with little apparent effort and fed it back in neat, professor-pleasing packages. He finished close enough to the top to win a scholarship to the Medical School of New York University. The scholarship was not quite enough to get him through his freshman year, and his parents had to borrow money. But he made the rest of the way on his own with scholarships.

Salk's academic performance at medical school was near the top, as expected, and the rest of the way —graduation, internship, and a successful practice— seemed to require no oracles for prediction. But before his freshman year at medical school was over, Salk, for the first time, did something that surprised and confounded his parents and peers. He decided that he did not want to become a practicing physician and announced to his incredulous parents that he wanted a research career. The times made Salk's decision even more difficult to understand. Salk started medical school in the mid-thirties when more Americans stood in bread lines than in registration lines at universities. For Salk there was hope, when for most men there was hopelessness, and his discarding of the promise of an independent practice for a salaried research job was more than anyone could understand.

Salk was adamant, and he demonstrated his seriousness by taking a year off from medical school to study biochemistry. To his parents this move must have seemed the most extreme of follies, for if he finally came to his senses and became a proper doctor with a shingle and an office he would have wasted a whole year. When Salk returned to medical school in 1936 he decided that bacteriology interested him most, and he devoted as much time as possible to his chosen field and still collected his usual "A's" in the regular courses.

Salk arranged to work with Thomas Francis, one of the better-known bacteriologists of the time. Francis had come to New York University from the Rockefeller Institute, where he had worked with Oswald Avery on the pneumococcus bacteria, one of the causes of pneumonia. Avery was later to become a well-known name to biology students as the result of some work he did with pneumococcus in 1944, along with two other American microbiologists, Colin M. MacLeod and Maclyn McCarty. The work done by this trio was a follow-up to some research done in 1929 by a British bacteriologist named Fred Griffith. Griffith had found that under certain circumstances a harmless variety of pneumococcus bacteria would somehow transform into a variety that could cause pneumonia. Avery and his co-workers, in a brilliant series of experiments, found that the "transforming substance" was deoxyribonucleic acid (DNA). This work pointed the way to later research, which eventually showed that DNA was the hereditary substance—that is, the material of which the gene is made.

Francis was not particularly interested in genetics, but he was interested in problems of immunity. Some of his ideas were considered to be unorthodox and, by many, even heretical. His belief that dead-virus vaccines were just as feasible as dead-bacteria vaccines was the heresy that earned for him the enmity of many of the old-line virologists.

Francis was born in Indiana in 1900, the son of a Methodist minister who was also a sometime steel worker. His family moved to Pennsylvania, and Francis went to Allegheny College in that state. During World War I he served in the Student Army Training Corps, and while the flu pandemic was raging he worked in hospital details. It was at this time that he decided on medicine as a career, and he developed a lifelong interest in influenza.

He graduated from Yale Medical School in 1925 and remained there through the steps of intern, resident, and instructor, so distinguishing himself that he was invited to join the Rockefeller Institute's hospital in 1928. He was eventually put in charge of influenza research in the Rockefeller Foundation's International

Health Division. When in 1933 influenza was definitely established as a viral disease, Francis naturally became interested in viruses. Among other things, he isolated new strains of flu virus and started to think about dead-virus vaccines.

Virology was a relatively new science in the 1930s and there were not too many full-time virologists. Most were primarily bacteriologists who considered the study of viruses as an extension of bacteriology. Virology was not considered to be a field with much of a future, and there were still some biologists who thought that viruses were not quite real. The few full-time virologists who were around jealously defended the little they knew or thought they knew about viruses, and they were, understandably, a rather insecure group of people. They resisted any new ideas that might undermine the treasured theories on which they had built careers.

So little was known about viruses that it was even a point of controversy to refer to them as organisms. The word "organism" means "living thing," and it was not at all clear that viruses were alive. Some virologists thought that viruses might be nothing more than fantastically small bacteria. Others thought that viruses were some kind of poisonous liquid.

The first hint of the existence of viruses had come in the 1890s with the work of Martinus Beijerinck in Holland and Dmitri Iwanowski in Russia. Both men worked independently with a disease of tobacco plants called the tobacco mosaic disease. While their work and their results were remarkably similar, the credit is usually given to Iwanowski alone. They both managed to extract from tobacco leaves a fluid that apparently contained the disease organism. They passed the fluid through a very fine porcelain filter with apertures small enough to prevent the passage of the smallest known bacteria. Whatever it was that caused the tobacco mosaic disease passed right through the filter, and for that reason the disease-causing substance was called a "filterable virus." The word "virus" means "poison," and for years it was used to denote anything bad, nasty, foul, or noxious. Pasteur had used the term "virus" to describe the cause of rabies, and that rabies is indeed caused by something that fits the present-day definition of viruses is somewhat of a coincidence.

Iwanowski published his results in 1892 and Beijerinck in 1898, and their work set off the first of many controversies about viruses. Were viruses actually particles like bacteria, only much smaller, or were viruses liquid and nothing but liquid? The latter question was answered to some degree in 1931 when William Elford, a microbiologist at the National Institute for Medical Research in England, designed a filter with pores small enough to trap the elusive viruses. His work seemed to indicate that viruses were indeed particulate, but investigators still did not know what viruses really were. (The electron microscope, which would enable scientists to see viruses, was still many years away.)

Wendell Stanley, an American biochemist, carried isolation to a new refinement in 1935, and in the wake of his work viruses seemed to be more enigmatic than ever. Stanley worked with the familiar tobacco mosaic disease virus (TMV). From about a ton of infected to-

bacco leaves, he laboriously extracted about a table-
spoonful of a white crystalline powder. The powder appeared to be no more alive than a spoonful of table
salt, but it was the virus. When the powder was
rubbed on a tobacco leaf, the symptoms of the disease
were soon apparent. The powder was many times more
infective than the liquid suspensions of the virus extracted by previous workers. It appeared that viruses
were on the borderline between the living and the
non-living. They assumed the properties of living
things only when they were inside a living cell. When
outside a living cell, viruses could crystallize in the
manner of inorganic salts.

Stanley's work indicated that viruses were not just
tiny bacteria but were something else that was very
strange indeed. Many more scientists became interested in viruses, and in the 1940s virology became a
fast-growing science. Eventually two basic schools
emerged: one was concerned with the diseases viruses
might cause and the related problems of immunity; the
other, with investigating viruses from the strictly biological point of view—that viruses were interesting
and deserved to be investigated for their own sake.

There was not a great deal of cooperation between
the two groups, and there was even some animosity.
Investigators interested in viral diseases tended, for the
most part, to be M.D.'s, and the biologists were Ph.D.'s.
Research physicians had a tendency to denigrate their
Ph.D. counterparts for "lack of concern with human-
ity," and biologists took pride in persuading promising
biology majors to go into pure biological research
rather than medicine.

Despite the rivalry, the two schools of research did complement each other. The biologists showed the doctors what viruses really were, and how they worked, and the M.D.'s, in their immunological work, uncovered some information on the chemical nature of viruses.

By the mid-1930s a little more was known about viruses than had been known at the beginning of the century, but not much more. It was known that they were very small, were perhaps alive and perhaps not. They would not grow on any of the usual growth media used for bacteria. Drugs were not effective against viral diseases, and doctors, then as now, could offer only the usual advice given for the common cold. Only three viral diseases—smallpox, rabies, and yellow fever—yielded to vaccines, and only the smallpox vaccine was widely used. All three were live-virus vaccines.

That one could acquire immunity to smallpox had been known a long time. Hundreds of years before Edward Jenner, an English physician of the late eighteenth century, observed that milkmaids who had had cowpox generally stayed healthy during smallpox epidemics, people knew that survivors of smallpox usually did not get the disease in subsequent epidemics. Out of these observations grew the practice of ingrafting, which involved scratching material from the sores of smallpox victims into healthy individuals. It was considered prudent to select a victim with a mild case, and many people with mild cases of smallpox sold the pustular products of their disease. Of course, no one knew why ingrafting worked. Indeed, it did not always work, and the result was sometimes a fatal case of smallpox rather than immunity. Primarily because of the uncertain nature of ingrafting, the practice fell into disfavor.

When Jenner experimented with cowpox pustules scratched into the arm of James Phipps in 1796, he based his hopes for success on the observation of the milkmaid phenomenon. The idea worked, but Jenner never knew why. Nor did he have any idea of what caused smallpox or what was in the cowpox pustules that induced immunity. Jenner's work, however, did help to establish the basic principle of induced immunity, and it provided us with the words "vaccination" and "vaccine" (which come from *vacca*, the Latin word for "cow").

Smallpox vaccination, which involves scratching some cowpox, or vaccinia virus, into the skin of the recipient, is a happy exception to the general rule that vaccines must be made from the specific organism that causes the disease in question.

The method of inducing immunity to rabies developed by Pasteur in 1885 did not really serve as a lasting answer because it was so dangerous and unsure that it was used only on people who had been bitten by rabid animals and were sure to die unless they received the Pasteur treatment. The rabies vaccine was dangerous because of the way it was made. Rabies virus was injected into the spinal cord of a rabbit. After a lapse of time, to give the virus a chance to grow, the spinal cord of the rabbit was ground up and the material injected into the spinal cord of another rabbit. The spinal cord of the second rabbit was then ground up and injected into the spinal cord of a third rabbit, and so on. This process served to weaken or "attenuate" the virus to the point where it would, hopefully, induce immunity but not cause the disease. Complications arose from the near impossibility of separating all the bits of spinal cord from the weakened virus. These bits of nervous tissue could cause a fatal encephalitis, an inflammation of the brain. But even that was better than the other possible complication of contracting rabies from some unweakened virus that might have survived the attenuation process. The decision to use rabies vaccine was particularly difficult in "bite and run" cases, where it was not known if the biting animal was rabid.

Since rabies vaccine is used on people only after the victim has been exposed to rabies, it is sometimes erroneously referred to as a "cure." It is not really a cure but a special case of inducing immunity. The after-the-bite immunity is made possible by the fact that the virus causes rabies only when it gets into the brain cells of the victim. The virus travels along the nervous system to the brain, a trip that takes from days to months depending upon how far away the bite is from the brain. An individual bitten on the toe has a long time to receive injections and to develop immunity before the virus reaches the brain.

Pasteur never knew just what caused rabies, but he assumed that it was caused by something so small that it could not be seen with a microscope. The virus of rabies was not identified until 1903. The vaccine used today to immunize dogs is made from virus grown and attenuated in chick embryos.

In 1908, Karl Landsteiner (the famous Viennese

scientist known for his work on blood groups) determined that a filterable virus was the cause of polio. Since paralytic polio is a disease of the nervous system, it was almost immediately assumed that the polio virus traveled along the nervous system in the same way as the rabies virus. This assumption led to one of the more bizarre attempts at control of polio. It was thought that the virus entered through the nose and traveled along the olfactory nerves to the brain. Dr. Edwin Schultz, a microbiologist at Stanford University, suggested that if a substance that would prevent the passage of the virus were sprayed into human noses, the prevention of polio could be the result. Dr. Schultz selected zinc sulfate because it was observed to cause coagulation of certain proteins in the mucus membranes of the nasal passage. So, in 1937, zinc-sulfate solution was sprayed into the noses of several thousand people, mostly children, during an epidemic of polio in Toronto. The only demonstrable result was that several of the recipients permanently lost their sense of smell. The belief that polio virus traveled along the nervous system persisted.

Mostly as a result of the Kolmer and Brodie vaccine disasters of 1935 polio immunology was not considered to be a particularly promising area of investigation. One of the major problems was the difficulty of culturing viruses. In order to make any kind of vaccine, bacterial or viral, dead or alive, large quantities of the disease organism are needed. Bacteria grow quite well in various nutrient broths and other media. Viruses, however, grow only in living cells, either in whole, live organisms or in cell and tissue cultures.

As early as the 1860s some biologists had devised methods of keeping excised cells and tissues alive in laboratory containers, that is, *in vitro*, which literally means "in glass." By the 1930s cell-culture techniques were fairly well advanced, but investigators were hampered by unwanted bacteria, which grew handily in the cell cultures. (This problem was not to be effectively handled until the development of antibiotics.) For the most part, polio virus was grown in live monkeys. There had been some limited success with growing polio virus in cell cultures, but it was widely accepted that polio virus would grow only in nerve cells.

This belief was fortified by a series of careful experiments carried out at the Rockefeller Institute in 1935 by Albert Sabin and Peter Olitsky, a leading American virologist of the time. They prepared cultures of various kinds of cells that had been removed from a still-born embryo and tried to grow polio viruses in the different cultures. Their polio virus flourished in nerve cells but not in kidney, liver, skin, or any other kind of cells.

The Sabin-Olitsky finding seemed to doom forever the hopes of making a polio vaccine. There seemed to be no way of culturing polio virus in sufficient quantities except in nerve-cell cultures or the spinal cords and brains of monkeys—and the dangers of contracting encephalitis from bits of nervous tissue were well known. It was one thing to inject a dangerous nervous-tissue-grown vaccine into the occasional victim of a mad dog bite who was going to die anyway, and quite another to inject hundreds of thousands of healthy people with a potentially death-dealing substance on the chance that it might induce immunity.

A number of people had tried to make flu vaccines, both live and inactive. None of these efforts was particularly successful, and the annoying tendency of flu viruses to mutate increased the virologists' frustration.

Small wonder, then, that many of the old-line virologists considered Francis a brash upstart for even thinking about trying to make a vaccine out of dead influenza virus. Various inactivated *bacterial* vaccines were very effective, but viruses were considered to be rather special, and the prevailing opinion was that inactivated-virus vaccines just would not work. But attempting to make a dead influenza-virus vaccine was exactly what Francis was doing when Salk came to work with him. Francis cultured influenza virus in cultures of minced chick embryos. When the virus was extracted it was irradiated with ultraviolet light, which hopefully killed the virus but not its ability to induce immunity. The work was inconclusive.

Francis soon left New York University and went to the University of Michigan. Salk, after graduation, interned at Mount Sinai Hospital in New York, where he again put in his usual brilliant performance, and when he was done he looked around for a research position. (He was not offered a position at Mount Sinai, since Mount Sinai interns were never offered jobs there.) When Salk applied to some of the more prestigious New York research institutions, he found that his long string of academic honors was not enough to get him a research job in New York City. Francis came to the aid of his former student.

At Michigan Francis's work on influenza vaccines was supported by the National Research Council on a grant from the National Foundation for Infantile Paralysis. Influenza was not polio, but both diseases were caused by viruses, and the directors of the foundation made many grants to researchers who were not working directly with polio but whose work might possibly be of some long-range benefit in the specific problem of polio. Francis managed to get an additional grant, which enabled Salk to join him at Michigan at a salary of $2400 a year.

Salk, although certainly disappointed by the rejections in New York, had much to look forward to in further work with Francis. During their previous association Salk too had become intrigued with the possibilities of killed-virus vaccines, and affiliation with Francis would enable him to pursue these interests further.

World War II had started when Salk went to Michigan. The Army was particularly interested in an effective influenza vaccine and provided Francis with more money. During the influenza pandemic of World War I and the immediate postwar years, 44,000 soldiers had died from influenza, and the Army was determined not to let this happen again.

The Army was not willing to take a chance on a live-virus vaccine, which could possibly revert to virulence and start an epidemic in the crowded conditions of an army base. Francis, with many years of experience in working with killed-virus vaccines, was a natural choice for this project. Francis tried different methods at Michigan; rather than using ultraviolet light, which had given indifferent results, Francis and Salk tried killing the viruses with formalin. (Brodie had tried the same thing with polio virus in 1935.) The idea was to determine how much formalin was just enough to kill the virus without impairing its ability to induce the body to form antibodies against it.

Another problem was the selection of viruses. The collection of symptoms commonly called influenza is not caused by one kind of virus but by several. Different kinds of viruses are called "types," a term that, when applied to viruses, is roughly akin to "species" as applied to ordinary organisms. Although different types of viruses may cause the same fever, muscle pain, and so on, as influenza, the types may be as different as a tiger and a house cat. Many of the previous attempts to prepare influenza vaccines had not been very successful because the early vaccines were made from only one type of virus and any conferred immunity was only against that type. Francis and the Army agreed that the best strategy was to make a vaccine from viruses considered to be the most prevalent types involved in influenza.

Choosing the right types was only part of the selection problem. Just as there are breeds of dogs within the species *Canis familiaris*, so are there different "breeds" of viruses within a type, and these are called "strains." A vaccine made from any strain of a type will usually confer immunity against all strains within the type if the vaccine is effective at all. The difficulty is that strains, as with breeds of dogs, have their own little peculiarities and characteristics. One strain may be more virulent than another—that is, more likely to cause disease. A vaccine made from a virulent strain is a lot more likely to confer stronger immunity than a less virulent one but may not be as safe—it might cause the disease instead of preventing it.

Stability was another characteristic that the early vaccine-makers desired for their virus strains but was not easy to obtain. A strain might exhibit good antigenicity (that is, stimulate the body to produce antibodies) and low virulence in trial after trial only to revert to virulence when injected as a vaccine. The basic problem was to find strains that would strike a balance between effectiveness and safety. For immunologists such as Francis and Salk, the process of choosing the most desirable strains was much like a guessing game, since strains of influenza virus were notoriously unstable and histories of infection were of little help.

Virologists tend to have favorite strains, and discussions of the merits of various strains sound much like "my dog is better than your dog." While types of viruses are generally designated by letters or Roman numerals, strains generally have more imaginative names. A strain may be named after the scientist who first isolated it, the place where it was isolated, or even after the individual human or animal from whom the virus was extracted.

By 1942 Francis had developed a killed-virus flu vaccine that incorporated strains of two types of viruses. He conducted field trials at army bases in 1942 and 1943, upon which he imposed a very stringent control system. One group received real vaccine and another group received a placebo—an inactive preparation that looked like the vaccine, and even stung like the vaccine when injected. Neither the injector nor the person receiving the shot nor the research team supervising the trials knew which was which. The injected materials were designated by a code, which was not broken until the trials were over. The trials were arranged this way to avoid prejudice in determining the results, for the scientist, like anyone else, tends to try to make things come out the way he thinks they should.

The 1942 trials were inconclusive since there was no epidemic that year. There was an epidemic in 1943, and the vaccine proved to be about 70 per cent effective. Thereafter the vaccine was in general use throughout the war years and was made available to civilians.

Francis and Salk knew that such vaccines were not likely to confer immunity as long-lasting as live-virus vaccines. They found that it was necessary to give booster shots at intervals as the immunity conferred by the killed-virus vaccine wore off. But that was all right with the Army; the soldiers were always available to get their shots when they needed them and they had little to say in the matter.

The two virologists published many papers together and sometimes Salk even had his name listed first. The question of whose name is listed first on a publication may seem a trifling matter, but it is as important to a scientist as top billing on a theater marquee to an actor. The implication is that the first-named author has made the most important and greatest contribution to the work even if that is not necessarily the case. After a while professional jealousies began to taint the relationship between the two men. Salk's slow rate of advancement at Michigan—by 1946 he was only an assistant professor—made him restless, and he began to look around for a situation where he would be free to do whatever research interested him.

In 1947 he accepted a position at the University of Pittsburgh Medical School. His title was virologist, and he was the only virologist there. In point of fact, he was not only the sole research worker but also the only full-time faculty member. At the time the University of Pittsburgh Medical School was considered to be a second-rate institution, located in one of the grimiest and dirtiest cities in North America. People were not as aware of environmental problems then, and the smoke-stacks of Pittsburgh's steel mills poured black smoke into the air unimpeded by any effective cry of protest.

Salk went to Pittsburgh because he thought that as the only full-time faculty member he would have his own way in choosing research projects. He found no utopia in grimy Pittsburgh. He was not at all his own boss and, since the university hospital was partly tax-supported, he had to beg all kinds of approvals and permissions from a bewildering array of city and university officials even to replace a broken test tube. Pittsburgh seemed like the end of the road to nowhere.

THE
END
OF
ORTHODOXY

AT THE END OF WORLD WAR II THE men on the board of the National Foundation for Infantile Paralysis found themselves confused and without direction. Although fund-raising campaigns continued during the war years, the major attention of the public was, naturally, on the events of the war and not on the publicity tactics of Basil O'Connor. With the death of Franklin Roosevelt in April 1945, the foundation had lost its big symbol but still had his memory to exploit. Research specifically relevant to the polio problem had lagged during the war, and the foundation people were not quite sure just how to start things up again to their best advantage.

The foundation had been generous with grants, and several institutions such as the Johns Hopkins

School of Public Health had received long-term grants of five years or more that totaled well into the millions of dollars. Rivers and others had convinced O'Connor that supporting basic research in virology was the best approach, and quite a bit of work not immediately relevant to polio was made possible by foundation dollars. The work of Francis on influenza was one example, and work on the epidemiology of equine encephalitis was another. Among biological scientists, especially virologists, the foundation came to be known as a ready source of grant money, which benefited the scientists as well as the scientific establishments. Moreover the Virus Research Committee of the foundation never pressured researchers to follow particular lines of research. On occasion Rivers may have suggested to a virologist that if he wanted to investigate something in particular the foundation just might support him and there would be nothing to lose in submitting a proposal.

Much of the polio work supported by the foundation between 1938 and 1947 was in the epidemiology and pathology of polio (and in nutrition studies, which later proved to lead nowhere in relationship to polio). The epidemiologists tried to determine how the disease was spread, and the pathologists were concerned with the effects of the virus on tissues. There were also quite a few fruitless efforts to find some kind of chemical cure.

The work of the epidemiologists and pathologists resulted in findings that should have overthrown some of the most dearly cherished polio orthodoxies. That they did not immediately do so was partly because the work was scattered and communication among virologists was poor; and mainly because orthodoxies have a way of growing long roots.

As early as the 1930s the recovery of polio virus in human stool samples had indicated that polio might be an intestinal disease and only incidentally a neurological affliction. Large amounts of virus had been recovered from the stools of people with non-paralytic polio, and since viruses grew only in living cells the polio virus must have grown in the cells of the intestine. Despite such findings, the dogma that polio virus grew only in nerve cells persisted. Belief that polio virus entered through the nose and traveled along the olfactory nerves to the brain also persisted despite pathological work by Sabin and others that revealed no lesions of the olfactory nerve in autopsies of polio victims. The few instances in which workers reported detecting polio virus in the bloodstream were ignored or dismissed as examples of sloppy work.

The strategy of waiting for assorted bacteriologists, physiologists, virologists, and epidemiologists to develop concepts and techniques that would collectively eliminate polio from the scene had not been very effective. By the mid-1940s the dream of a vaccine or cure was no closer to becoming a reality than it had been in 1935. So, in the immediate postwar years, O'Connor faced a rather dismal prospect. The orthodox virologists continued to preach that a safe vaccine was out of the question because polio virus would grow only in nervous tissue and no vaccine made from virus grown in nerve cells was safe. They also maintained that since polio virus traveled along nerves and not in the blood, large amounts of that unsafe vaccine would have to be injected if any of it was to get at the virus in the nervous system.

Meanwhile the number of polio cases was increasing, and money was needed to take care of the victims in addition to money needed for research. The "significant breakthroughs" upon which the foundation fundraisers relied to inspire the public to greater giving were non-existent. The foundation still depended on the public for its sustenance, and the public was fickle. A fair amount of money was still collected, but much of it was from habitual givers, those people who automatically deposited their change in the little boxes that bore the pathetic pictures of paralyzed children in braces and wheelchairs. Giving money to conquer polio was the thing to do; it was part of the mother-and-the-flag national mystique, and not to give was considered somewhat "unpatriotic."

O'Connor was well aware that even this trickle of dimes and quarters could dry up if something exciting did not happen soon. He had always relied on press releases that contained such phrases as "encouraging development" to keep the public in a giving mood even though he ran the risk of receiving angry letters from embarrassed scientists. O'Connor assumed even more risk of angering scientists when, in 1946, a semi-retired virologist, Harry Weaver, was appointed Director of Research in an attempt to launch a concerted research effort. The risk to O'Connor lay in what was implied in Weaver's title. Scientists have never liked to be directed, but O'Connor felt that he had waited long enough for scientists to eliminate polio with their individual, uncoordinated efforts. Direction was needed, engineered in such a way that the independent-minded scientists would not know they were being directed. That was Harry Weaver's job.

Weaver began by organizing a series of meetings of foundation grantees, the ostensible purpose of which was to facilitate communications among the various workers. This certainly happened, but the real purpose was to acquaint Harry Weaver with the state of polio research and to provide him with a starting point for his direction.

Through some two years of meetings about virus research, Weaver learned much, and in his position of observer, with no pet theories of his own to defend, he was able to see a few things that the entrenched virologists could not or would not see. He was impressed with evidence, some of it dating back to the turn of the century, that the usual abode of the polio virus was the intestine and not the nervous system. In memos to Rivers and O'Connor he expressed his deep concern with the tendency of established virologists to cling to such beliefs as the exclusively neurotrophic nature of polio virus in the face of strong evidence to the contrary. He found that the alleged neurotropic property of polio virus was an effective barrier even to the consideration of a vaccine. Because of the danger of encephalitis no one in his right mind would propose the injection of a vaccine made of virus grown on nervous tissue. This wall of doubt built by the older generation of virologists was at last brought down, brick by brick, by the work that was being done by younger people. The way to what O'Connor would later call a "planned miracle" was open.

The Johns Hopkins School of Public Health and Hygiene had long been one of the biggest beneficiaries of foundation largesse. In 1941 Kenneth Maxcy, a Johns Hopkins classmate of Rivers, had proposed to the foundation that a permanent research center be set up at Hopkins. An initial grant of $300,000 for a period of five years was made in 1942. The center was not to limit its activities to polio but was also to investigate other virus diseases. Maxcy, as director, had complete authority. The grant was as much a coup for the foundation as it was for Johns Hopkins, for up to that point most virus work there had been supported by a rival philanthropy called the Commonwealth Fund.

Maxcy assembled some of the best young virologist talent in the country, if not the world. Among them were David Bodian, Howard Howe, and Isabel Morgan. The findings issued from this group soon had the orthodox virologists running for cover.

David Bodian was one of those rare savants who, as a Ph.D. and M.D., could approach research problems without yielding to the philosophical prejudices of either of the two academic schools. He was trained as an anatomist and was regarded as an expert neurologist. He had been at Johns Hopkins since 1939 and had done some work on polio pathology with Howard Howe, as grantees of the Commonwealth Fund. Howe was also at Hopkins as an associate in the anatomy department of the medical school.

Isabel Morgan came from a family in which science was a way of life. Her father was Thomas Hunt Morgan, senior member of the fabled "Drosophila group" of Columbia University which established much of the body of knowledge of classical genetics through work with the fruit fly called *Drosophila*. After obtaining a Ph.D. in bacteriology at the University of Pennsylvania she worked at the Rockefeller Institute with Peter Olitsky on inactivated-virus vaccines for encephalomyelitis. She also did a little work with polio viruses. In 1944 she joined Bodian and Howe.

Bodian, Howe, and Morgan attempted to immunize monkeys with inactivated polio virus preparations similar to those made by Brodie in 1935. On some occasions these monkeys survived challenges with live polio virus and at other times they did not. This work not only pointed to possibilities of killed-virus polio vaccines but also indicated that there was probably more than one type of polio virus. Further work suggested that there were three types of polio virus, but neither the Johns Hopkins group nor anyone else could be absolutely sure of this. There could be four, or five, or twenty-seven types for that matter.

The evidence for the existence of different types of polio virus was not particularly startling. That there were different types of viruses involved in other diseases was widely known, and also that different types of viruses could cause essentially the same disease. Francis was certainly well aware of this from his years of frustration trying to make a vaccine that would be effective against all viruses that cause what we call influenza. What was apparent to all, now, was one of the reasons for the failure of the Kolmer and Brodie vaccines. They had used only one type of virus in their vaccine preparations, in addition to using sloppy techniques in the over-all preparation. It was clear that any proposed polio vaccine would have to be effective against all types of polio virus.

Before a truly effective polio vaccine could be considered to be even a remote possibility, all the known strains of polio viruses had to be typed to determine if there were indeed only three types. Typing viruses was not particularly exciting work. It was the kind of job usually given to a graduate assistant or to a technician. A virologist who thought much of himself was not likely to volunteer to spend several years running typing tests on literally thousands of known polio strains, not to mention the new ones that kept cropping up. Typing viruses was dull, tedious work and not the stuff of which Nobel Prizes were made.

It was Harry Weaver's job to convince one or more young virologists that typing viruses was indeed an exciting thing to do. He concentrated his efforts on contacting young, relatively unknown men. He knew without asking that any established virologist would consider such drudgery and tedium beneath his dignity. Equally important in Weaver's search were institutional facilities. The typing project would require large numbers of monkeys—and a great deal of space is needed to keep monkeys.

One of the men who came to Weaver's attention was Jonas Salk, who was working on flu virus at Pittsburgh. Salk had no experience with polio virus, but that was good, since he was less likely to be encumbered with orthodox notions. Even better was the facility at Salk's disposal. With the advent of antibiotics, the old contagious disease wards in the university hospital were empty. Salk had wanted this space but had been unable to convince the hospital trustees that he could put the space to good use. But it was available, and Weaver knew it.

Salk eagerly accepted Weaver's suggestion, and the university and city officials agreed to donate the use of the empty wards. Weaver was also successful in persuading virologists in Kansas, Utah, and California to do some typing work.

The foundation, noted for its propensity for gathering committees, duly organized a Typing Committee to oversee the work of Salk and the others. The committee was made up of many of the major figures in virology, such as Albert Sabin, Thomas Francis, David Bodian, John Paul, and William Hammon, the men who would not give any of their own time to the actual typing. As members of the committee, they understood that their job was to tell the virus typers how to do their work. It was further understood that Salk and the others would do exactly as they were told. (It seems that Weaver did not make that absolutely clear when he did his persuading.) The Typing Committee eventually became the Immunization Committee.

Preparations for the big project took over a year to complete and the actual work did not begin until 1949. Salk had a particular problem. The empty wards needed much remodeling to convert them into laboratories, and the grant did not cover this. The local foundation chapter offered to use its own March of Dimes money to pay for the necessary carpentry, electrical wiring, plumbing, and so forth. This, however, was definitely against the rules, for according to the by-laws of the foundation only the duly designated committees at the national office could make grants. O'Connor, who thought the hospital should be responsible for the carpentry, was livid at the Pittsburgh rebellion, and Salk was caught in the middle. The impasse was broken when a local charity not connected with the foundation donated the money.

As the project wore on, Salk found that he had less and less time to spend in the laboratory, for more and more time was required at his desk. He had to attend to problems of budget, acquiring supplies, and renewing grants. (The ascendancy of the desk over the laboratory bench is still a problem confronting many scientists.)

At times he was little more than a monkey-keeper. Monkeys were a mainstay of polio research. At the time they were the only known, readily available animal susceptible to all types of polio, and that was unfortunate for polio researchers. Monkeys were expensive to buy, difficult to maintain, and took up a great deal of room in the laboratory. They were much more difficult to handle than the duller rabbits and mice. Monkeys, nasty-tempered, especially the widely used Rhesus monkey, could inflict vicious bites. In 1935 a promising young bacteriologist, William Brebner, was bitten by a monkey and died of a paralytic disease. The cause of death was determined to be a previously unknown virus, which was called the B virus in honor of Dr. Brebner. The B virus was isolated and identified by Albert Sabin, who had just started at the Rockefeller Institute.

In captivity, the habits of monkeys cannot be described as clean, and housebreaking is an unknown concept in connection with them. They have a rather disconcerting habit of defecating into their hands and throwing the excrement at passers-by. Any qualms at the "inhumanity" of injecting viruses into the spinal cords of these "cute" creatures, who look so much like little people, is soon dispelled by their many annoying attributes.

The monkeys had to be imported from Southeast Asia, and many of them died from respiratory ailments in transit or shortly after arrival. It was frequently necessary to expend time and money in nursing the animals back to health before they could be used. There were so many casualties that the foundation decided to go into the monkey business. A monkey farm was set up in South Carolina, and this operation supplied polio researchers with most of the monkeys they needed.

The accepted method of testing the virus strains was laborious and very expensive in terms of time and the number of monkeys that had to be sacrificed. A researcher would start with a strain of a known type, say, Type I. A number of monkeys would be injected with the Type I virus, and those that survived would be assumed to be immune to Type I. Then an unknown strain would be injected into the Type I-immune monkeys. If the animals survived, the unknown virus was known to be Type I. If the monkey got polio, then the unknown strain had to be Type II or Type III. If that was the case, the procedure was repeated with monkeys previously determined to be immune to Types II and III. The procedure required a huge supply of monkeys, and the result was far from certain. Some strains were more infectious than others, and it was entirely possible that a given monkey might succumb to one strain of virus but not to another strain within the same type. Some economy was made possible when it was found that some Type II strains would infect mice. These animals could be used to determine if an unknown strain was Type II, and since mice were much cheaper than monkeys, the savings were considerable.

At meetings various proposals were made to the Typing Committee to modify the procedure in the interest of saving time and monkeys—that is, money. Several workers had noted that polio antibodies could be recovered from the blood serum of previously uninfected monkeys that had been injected with polio virus. This was the case whether the monkey died, survived, or did not come down with polio at all. It was therefore proposed that the typing be done by injecting the unknown strain into a healthy monkey first. Then the blood of the monkey would be checked against samples of each of the known virus types to see which sample was neutralized by the antibodies in the monkey's blood. This was proposed as more than a great time-and-monkey saver. It was suspected that some strains existed that were too weak to cause infection but could still induce antibody formation. A procedure that depended on infecting monkeys would not be very useful in typing these strains. These proposals were rejected by the virologist establishment that made up the Typing Committee, and it was made very clear that the typers were to do as they were told.

The Typing Committee was very much concerned with setting standards to be adhered to by all workers in the typing project. There was concern that, if each of the typers did his own thing in his own way, controls would be non-existent and no meaningful results would be obtained. On the other hand, the function of the typing project was to type viruses, and it would seem that the method was secondary as long as the job was done.

The methods proposed by the younger workers seemed quite sensible in view of the fact that polio antibodies had been detected in the blood of thousands of people who had never had paralytic polio. However, the contention of many of the older virologists that these people had not harbored *enough* virus to cause infection was just as sensible as the arguments of the newcomers that some strains would not cause paralytic polio no matter how much was there, and that different people reacted to the virus in different ways. If the latter were the case, then such would certainly be the case in monkeys and therefore dependence on infecting monkeys was not at all sensible.

To some workers the presence of polio antibodies in the blood seemed to indicate that the portal of entry and the route of polio virus was not the nervous system. Yet the established virologists still clung to the idea that polio was a disease of the nervous system only, pointing out that to find actual polio virus in the blood of polio victims was a very rare thing. The tenacity of the old-liners was understandable. It was hard to part with ideas that had been companions for as long as half a century.

The actual work of typing viruses went very quickly, primarily because faster methods were adopted by many of the typers, notably Salk, in spite of the establishment's instructions. Salk was quickly bored with the mechanics of this work, and long before the project was finished he was looking for other things to do. That there would be other things to do in polio research was being determined at Johns Hopkins and in the Boston laboratory of John F. Enders, who happened to be annoyed with the virus that causes mumps.

John Enders is among the last of the vanishing breed of gentleman scientists (in the Age of Enlightenment sense). He was born into an established and wealthy New England family and could have done just about anything he wanted to do. Indeed, he tried many things before he became a virologist. In his life there was none of the intense upward struggle of Jonas Salk or the desperate poverty of Albert Sabin. He became a scientist because he thought it might be an interesting thing to do, and he took his time about it.

John Enders was born in West Hartford, Connecticut, in 1897, the son of a banker and the grandson of the president of the Aetna Insurance Company. He served as a flying instructor in World War I, went to Yale, and tried to sell real estate after his graduation in 1920. But he did not sell many houses, and he thought that perhaps he ought to try graduate school at Harvard. He spent four years in the gentlemanly pursuit of English literature and Celtic and Teutonic languages before a roommate introduced him to the bacteriolo-

gist Hans Zinsser. What Zinsser was doing seemed to
Enders a good deal more intriguing than his own prospect of teaching literature and languages. With his
thesis in English literature almost finished, Enders
changed course and took a Ph.D. in bacteriology. He
was to be one of the Ph.D.'s who showed the M.D. researchers the way to a polio vaccine.

He soon found viruses more to his liking than bacteria, and in his quiet, deliberate way he soon made a
reputation for himself in virology. He was particularly
interested in growing viruses in tissue cultures. During
the World War II years Enders started to work on a
mumps vaccine and, in collaboration with Joseph
Stokes, Jr., developed a killed-virus vaccine of moderate and temporary effectiveness. In the 1950s Stokes,
then at the University of Pennsylvania, was one of the
first to demonstrate that hepatitis could be transmitted
in transfused blood. The mumps vaccine was made
from virus grown in the salivary glands of monkeys,
since Enders had been unable to grow the virus in tissue culture, a circumstance that bothered him.

In 1946 Children's Hospital in Boston asked him
to set up a new infectious disease laboratory. One of
his first efforts there was a renewed effort to cultivate
the balky mumps virus in tissue culture. He was joined
in his efforts by Thomas H. Weller and Frederick C.
Robbins after their service in World War II; both were
graduates of Harvard Medical School. Their work was
indirectly supported by the National Foundation for
Infantile Paralysis, which had granted $200,000 to the
Harvard Bacteriology Department for a five-year virus
study. Some of this money was given to the Enders

group. As grants go, it was as penny candy compared to the lavish five-pound-box sums expended by the foundation. It was the biggest bargain the foundation ever bought.

By 1948 the Enders team was growing mumps virus in a tissue culture made primarily of chick-embryo pieces and ox blood. The problem of bacterial contamination was overcome with antibiotics. They also succeeded in growing mumps virus in a variety of human embryonic tissue obtained from stillborn babies. When the mumps experiments were done, Enders had a few tissue cultures left over and he was loath to throw them away. He had some "Lansing strain" polio virus in his freezer, and he was curious to see what would happen if he put this virus into his cultures of human embryonic skin and muscle tissue. The strain had been isolated from an eighteen-year-old boy who had died of polio in Lansing, Michigan. The polio virus grew in the tissue, and it was *not* nervous tissue.

The Enders team did not run to the Harvard Yard and proclaim their discovery. There were more questions to answer. Would polio virus grow in mature human tissue as well as embryonic? Was the Lansing strain's ability to grow in non-nervous tissue atypical? The first question was answered by growing the Lansing strain in foreskin tissue, chosen because of its availability from circumcisions. The answer to the latter question was the more important in terms of implications for vaccine-makers. Strains of the other two types were tried, and they grew very well in cultures of embryonic and mature *non-nervous* human tissue as well as in non-nervous monkey tissues.

Their experience was the reverse of what had happened to Sabin and Olitsky in 1935. They too had tried to grow polio virus in human tissue culture, but their strain had grown only in nervous tissue. The strain Sabin and Olitsky had used was atypical. It had become neurotropic as the result of repeated passage through the brains of laboratory animals. They had had no way of knowing this, and their choice of a virus was one of those unfortunate accidents of science. It would seem that Sabin and Olitsky should have tried other strains of virus, but at that time the idea that there were different types of polio virus had not yet surfaced. If Sabin and Olitsky had tried other strains, there might have been a polio vaccine fourteen years sooner.

Enders, Weller, and Robbins published their findings in *Science* on January 28, 1949, in an article entitled "Cultivation of the Lansing Strain of Poliomyelitis Virus in Cultures of Various Human Embryonic Tissues." It was not even a lead article: it was confined to a few columns in the back pages.

Enders was certainly aware of the significance of his work, that it made an effective polio vaccine only a matter of time. He was also aware of what the development of a vaccine would do to his privacy. He wanted no reporters, television cameras, or curiosity seekers swarming all over his laboratory. Nor did he have any desire to leave New England to make fund-raising speeches for the foundation. However, he did journey to Stockholm in 1954, in the company of Weller and Robbins, to accept a Nobel Prize for the virus culture work. In point of fact, he told the Nobel committee that he would not accept the prize unless it was shared with Weller and Robbins.

Amazingly, the work of the Enders group was accepted with hardly a murmur of dissent by the virologist community. Polio research entered an active new phase, in which even the old-liners joined, for orthodoxy was no longer fashionable.

Jonas Salk, caught up in the excitement generated by the work of Enders, Morgan, Bodian, and others, wanted to work on a polio vaccine, and so did many others. The Johns Hopkins group, particularly Howard Howe, was interested, and Sabin made no secret of his desire to be the latter-day Pasteur. Salk, Sabin, the Johns Hopkins people, and most of the country's virologists looked to the foundation for support, but none of the foundation-supported virologists started the vaccine race in first position.

Even before the revelations of Enders and Bodian, two virologists, Herald Cox and Hilary Koprowski, had been working on an attenuated vaccine. Their situation was much different from that of Salk and Sabin. They were in the employ of the Lederle Division of the American Cyanamid Company, one of the largest pharmaceutical manufacturers in the world, and their money and support came from the company. Their situation at Lederle was unique. Never before had a commercial enterprise so committed itself to the development of a vaccine from scratch. Usually a pharmaceutical concern would provide its resources for the manufacture of a vaccine or similar medication after the basic research had been done elsewhere.

Cox and Koprowski were definitely contenders for

vaccine honors, and the virologists who presented vaccine proposals to the foundation did so in the knowledge that the pair at Lederle could very well get there first. The competition was congenial enough—Cox and Koprowski often attended foundation-sponsored meetings on vaccine problems—but it was nonetheless a race, and the foundation did not want to be second. One of the remaining orthodoxies, the idea that the polio virus traveled along nerve fibers and was not found in the blood, was challenged by the results of the first of the foundation immunization programs. This was the gamma-globulin program, an idea that was proposed and rejected many times before the foundation spent a dime on it.

Globulins are blood proteins, and gamma globulin is one of those in which antibodies are formed. The techniques for separating blood into its various fractions, such as fibrinogens and globulins, were developed during World War II by Dr. Edwin Cohn at Harvard. The injection of gamma globulin does not stimulate the body to produce antibodies. The immunity induced by gamma globulin is passive—that is, the recipient makes use of the antibodies that are already present in the gamma globulin. The effect is temporary and wears away when the antibodies break down.

The possibilities of using gamma globulin in epidemics and during the summer polio "season" were seen by some workers as early as 1940. Dr. Sidney Kramer of the Michigan Department of Health made such a proposal to the foundation in 1941 but it was rejected. Even as early as 1930 blood serum from patients was injected into siblings of polio victims in an attempt to prevent the spread of the disease within a family. It seemed to work, but it had not been tested in a controlled experiment. (A single injection of the gamma globulin used in the foundation's program represented the blood of hundreds of donors and was much richer in antibodies than serum. It was also much more expensive.)

Other gamma-globulin proposals were made in the 1940s, but it was not until the early 1950s that the foundation was ready seriously to consider gamma-globulin experiments.

The orthodox virologists were skeptical because they could not see how an ordinary type of intramuscular injection could be very effective against a virus domiciled in the nervous system. It was thought that a rather large and consequently painful injection would be required to insure that enough antibody got to the nervous system. The expense of a gamma-globulin program, the temporary nature of the immunity, and the fact that the Red Cross, which ran the national blood program, was reluctant to supply the necessary amounts of gamma globulin, also contributed to the foundation's reluctance.

The rapid development of polio research following the work of Enders resulted in a change of attitude. Isabel Morgan's successful immunization of monkeys also contributed to the willingness of O'Connor to consider gamma globulin. Especially convincing was the work of Dr. Joseph Stokes, Jr., who demonstrated that a small amount of gamma globulin gave protection against infectious hepatitis. Stokes was one of the men who had proposed gamma globulin to the foundation and had been refused.

There remained much that was uncertain when the foundation approved a limited gamma-globulin field trial in 1951. The major problem was just how much gamma globulin would have to be injected. It was generally agreed that the dose would have to be below 10 cc. It is not the size of a needle that makes an intramuscular injection painful. Rather, it is the amount of liquid injected. Rivers felt that if word got around that the shot was painful, the subjects, particularly children, would go into hiding. It was believed by many virologists, however, that less than 10 cc would not be enough.

The individual who finally convinced the foundation to approve and finance a gamma-globulin field trial was William Hammon. Hammon, a virologist and epidemiologist, had worked with Enders in the preparation of a vaccine for cat distemper. He was the son of a missionary, and there was much of the missionary in his zeal for gamma globulin. According to many present at the meetings of the Immunization Committee that considered the proposal, the debate was ended and the project approved when Rivers said, "Let's throw scientific discussion out of the window and do the experiment." Rivers was not opposed to scientific discussion, but the fact was that nothing could be resolved in the meeting room and that consensus could come only from carrying out the experiment. There has always been some risk in medical procedures, but the risk here was low. Even if gamma globulin proved to be ineffective, there was little possibility of any harm resulting from the injections.

The first trial was carried out in Provo, Utah, in the late spring of 1951. Hammon divided the children into groups according to their weight and injected amounts from 4 cc to 10 cc accordingly. One group of children received gamma globulin and another received a placebo. The results were encouraging. The relatively small amounts raised the level of antibody in the blood, and only one case of polio occurred in the experiment group; several occurred in the placebo control group.

Larger field trials were conducted in 1952 in Houston, Texas, and Sioux City, Iowa. The immunity conferred was indeed temporary, about six weeks, but gamma globulin was seen as a means of protecting children during epidemics and over much of the summer polio season.

The results of the field trials impressed Bodian at Johns Hopkins. The effectiveness of the small dose of gamma globulin suggested that the polio virus must get to the nervous system via the bloodstream. So in 1952 Bodian and Dr. Dorothy Horstmann of Yale, working independently, began to look for polio virus in the blood of monkeys and chimpanzees. They fed virus to the animals and, a few days following the feedings, found polio virus in the blood. When the virus was detected the animals did not have paralytic polio, but later many of them did develop paralysis. The condition of virus in the blood is called "viremia." The last of the "unalterable" dogmas, that polio virus was never to be found in the blood, had fallen.

In the almost fifty years that polio had been known to be a viral disease, polio virus had been found in the blood of victims in only one or two isolated instances. The reason was, of course, that by the time paralytic symptoms were evident, the virus had left the bloodstream and had become established in the nervous system. The few observed viremias had been explained away as instances of the virus spilling over from the nervous system into the blood. Some orthodox virologists still tried to argue that this was the case in the work of Bodian and Horstmann, but the pieces fitted together too neatly. The old school had to give up at last. The large amounts of polio virus found in stool samples, the demonstration of viremia, and the success of gamma globulin, all indicated strongly that polio was a widespread intestinal infection that could get to the nervous system via the bloodstream.

The epidemiological work done by John Paul in 1946 did much to complete the picture. Paul had found an almost 100 per cent incidence of polio antibodies in the blood of Arab children in North Africa. These children lived in filth and squalor and few ever got paralytic polio. The answer was that the squalor of their surroundings insured exposure to polio virus when they still retained the antibodies obtained as fetuses or nursing babies. The mother's antibodies were able to penetrate the placental barrier, and these were enough to provide protection until the baby built its own antibodies. Paul found that the antibody level in American children was very low. It was now clear that if polio was to be eliminated in countries with high standards of living, the general polio-antibody level of the population had to be raised, not by squalor, but with vaccines.

The way to a vaccine was now open, and that its development would be financed by the foundation was not questioned. The question was, who was going to be the foundation's vaccine hero?

A
HERO
IS
CREATED

■■■■■■■■■■■■■■■■■■■■■■■■■■■■

SALK, IN 1949, WAS NOT AMONG THE virologist elite who took part in setting foundation policy. Perhaps because he thought that a lowly virus typer's proposal might be met with less than enthusiasm by the eminent figures on the Immunization Committee, he directed his first, tentative inquiries to Harry Weaver, who at first was not very encouraging.

Salk wanted to try Ender's tissue-culture techniques, but his foundation grant did not cover this. He looked to other sources, and the University of Pittsburgh managed to get him $7500, which was enough to buy some equipment and hire a technician. He begged some starter cultures from Enders, taught himself how to grow polio virus in tissue culture, and was soon using culture-grown viruses in the typing work.

Salk made no secret of the tissue-culture work, nor did he have to. Although the work was not sanctioned by the foundation, O'Connor made no comment, for he never made any attempt to control the outside activities of foundation grantees. What they did on their own time and with their own or someone else's money was none of O'Connor's business, as long as the work for which the foundation paid was done.

Not only did the foundation not interfere with Salk's tissue-culture work, it gave him more money when the modest university grant ran out. Salk and his staff became rather adept at tissue culture and developed techniques to grow virus in the testicular and kidney tissue of monkeys, which was more readily available than human tissues. He injected some of his cultivated viruses into monkeys and found that high antibody levels resulted. Salk still deployed his findings to the Weaver flank rather than directly to the Immunization Committee.

In June of 1950 Salk indicated to Weaver that he had progressed to the point where he was ready to make a formal proposal to the foundation. At this time he was not yet fully committed to a killed-virus vaccine injected into people. He was giving some thought to injecting hens and cows with a killed-virus preparation in the hope that antibodies would spill over into yolks and milk respectively. People, especially children, could then be passively immunized in the normal course of drinking milk and get a super load of antibodies from drinking eggnog. Perhaps he had adults in mind with the eggnog, although in his letters to Weaver he did not make this clear; nor did he say if what adults frequently put into eggnog would effect the antigenic qualities of the beverage. This would appear to be a rather odd approach to immunization, but its basis was sound, at least in theory. It had long been known that babies obtained antibodies from mother's milk. Polio virus was known by then to inhabit the intestine before it got to the nervous system, and the antibodies in the ingested milk and eggnog could possibly intercept the virus in the intestine, conferring a continuously renewed passive immunity.

Salk was still thinking of milk and eggs as a possibility when he presented his proposal to the foundation in July of 1950. He had already injected a number of cows and chickens with the killed viruses. The grant was awarded and left him open to explore active immunization as an alternative if nothing encouraging happened in the barnyard. There was nothing particularly momentous in the grant. The men of the foundation would have been overjoyed to empty their coffers for Enders or Francis as well, but these two made no vaccine proposals and nothing would persuade them to do so.

Thanks to Harry Weaver, polio researchers were better informed about the over-all picture than they had ever been before. Weaver accomplished this information exchange by holding frequent meetings. At one such meeting, held in Hershey, Pennsylvania (of chocolate-bar fame), in March 1951, Koprowski surprised everyone and angered many by announcing that he had fed some of his live, attenuated viruses—in chocolate milk—to a group of "volunteers." The volunteers were mentally defective children in an institution in

New York State, and it was obvious that the volunteering had been done for them. Rivers was particularly angered by this report. When Koprowski had requested permission to carry out the experiment, the New York authorities went to Rivers to seek his advice. Rivers unequivocally advised against the use of human subjects in polio experiments at that time, not only because it was dangerous but because it was unethical. Having assumed that his advice had been taken and that Koprowski had been refused permission, Rivers was doubly shocked.

At this same meeting Isabel Morgan reported on killed-virus experiments with monkeys, and Howard Howe reported on the same, except that he had used chimpanzees and his viruses had not been grown in tissue culture but in the spinal cord of monkeys. He too spoke of plans for human experimentation with his nerve-grown strains, much to the horror of many at the meeting.

Salk heard from some formidable competition. Sabin had yet to say anything about what he was doing.

The Second International Poliomyelitis Congress was held in Copenhagen in September 1951, and Salk was chosen by the Immunization Committee to speak on the virus-typing program. On the return trip, aboard the *Queen Mary*, Salk met Basil O'Connor. The impression that Salk made on O'Connor was definitely a factor in the foundation's decision to support Salk massively in his vaccine work and to take the gamble on a large field trial of the vaccine he was developing.

Salk had given up the idea of passive immunization and had begun to concentrate on a killed-virus vaccine, in which he had always had confidence. His concentration was perhaps disturbed somewhat by the appointment of William Hammon, of gamma-globulin fame, as professor of epidemiology at the University of Pittsburgh's Graduate School of Public Health. Reportedly, Salk had wanted the job, and he was apparently annoyed when someone else got it. Equally annoying was Hammon's zeal for gamma globulin, which was in direct opposition, in philosophy, to Salk's zeal for a killed-virus vaccine. Hammon sincerely felt that gamma globulin was the only way to accomplish mass polio immunization. He believed that while the individual enjoyed the passive, temporary immunity of gamma globulin, the body would have a chance actively to build its own antibodies if exposed to polio virus. Hammon was suspicious of anyone whose work might maneuver his gamma globulin out of favor.

Although Salk and Hammon were on the same university campus, mutual suspicion and jealousies kept them apart. This was unfortunate, for an exchange of ideas between the two men would certainly have been of benefit to the development of a good, safe polio preventative, which was, after all, the central issue.

The advent of gamma globulin had an effect on the tenor of vaccine work. Gamma globulin whetted the public's appetite for a polio preventative, and the publicity given the gamma-globulin field trials put pressure on Salk and the foundation to hurry. The foundation spent over $14,000,000 on the 1951 gamma-globulin program. Calculating from the approximate six weeks' immunity conferred by a shot, this came to a cost of almost $2,500,000 a week. Even the foundation, with its huge coffers of dimes, could not keep up this level of expenditure. But as long as there was nothing else available the foundation felt an obligation to continue gamma-globulin programs.

A predictable outcome of the gamma-globulin program was that everybody wanted it for his children, and an ugly black market could have developed if O'Connor had not bought up every available drop on the market. Worried parents still attempted to bribe and to use all available influence to get their children immunized. Emotions ran high, and many parents nurtured the fear that because they did not have the right connections their child might get polio and suffer paralysis or die.

Salk, once committed to a killed-virus vaccine, toyed with the idea of killing the virus with ultraviolet radiation but soon gave that up in favor of formalin. This was ominously reminiscent of the Brodie disaster of 1935 and raised some doubts among many virologists, including Enders and Sabin. Although Enders wanted nothing to do with developing vaccines, he believed that the only way to make a vaccine was with live, attenuated virus. Enders was reported to have referred to Salk's work as quackery.

Ultraviolet light never had worked in actual practice. Salk knew that from his work with Francis in 1938. Although Brodie had indeed used formalin, he had not known that there were different types of polio virus. If there was anything Salk was in a supreme position to know, it was that there were three types and many, many strains of polio virus.

One of the most difficult and crucial problems facing Salk was the choice of strains to be used in the vaccine. To be "best," a strain had to meet several qualifications. It had to grow well in tissue culture, well enough to produce a good harvest of virus. It had to possess sufficient virulence to induce antibody formation. The more virulent a strain, the more antibody formation it was likely to induce. On the other hand, the more virulent the strain, the more likely it was to cause the disease before it could induce immunity to the disease. A weak strain might be safe, but worthless if it did not induce antibody formation. As far as Salk was concerned, a very important characteristic was that it had to be readily killable but still capable of inducing immunity after it was killed.

Salk found strains for Type II and Type III with relative ease. The Type II virus was the MEF strain, which had been isolated from British troops in the Middle East Forces during World War II. Type III was represented by the so-called Saukett strain, which Salk had isolated from the stool of a paralyzed boy named James Sarkett. The label on the stool-sample container had been sloppily written and the r was read as a u. Once the misnomer had been published, it persisted in all the virology literature.

The choice of a Type I virus proved to be particularly difficult. This was unfortunate because Type I polio was the most prevalent form of the disease. Strains that grew well in culture either were too weak

or too difficult to kill; strains that were good antibody
producers would not yield good tissue-culture harvests.
Other strains grew well in culture but were considered
to be dangerous. A Type I strain with an ideal set of
characteristics seemed not to exist.

After months of searching for the ideal Type I
strain Salk decided that the most important factor was
really the strain's antigenic properties. He reasoned
that no matter how virulent a strain was in nature,
once it was killed it was killed; however virulent, it
would be killed if exposed to the killing agent long
enough. He reasoned further that virulence was a desirable characteristic since the more virulent it was, the
more antigenic it was. He therefore chose the highly
virulent Mahoney strain, isolated from a family in
Ohio, for his Type I virus. The Mahoney strain had a
very nasty reputation, and rightfully so, for, although
the Mahoney family came through the illness, the children in the house next door were all paralyzed.

Despite warnings and misgivings from his colleagues, Salk committed himself to the Mahoney strain
as the only acceptable Type I virus. He may have felt
some apprehension about his choice but was rather
pleased that his Type I was highly antigenic and flourished in monkey kidney tissue.

Basically Salk had three variables to consider:
temperature, time, and the proportion of virus to formalin. Largely through trial and error, he surmised
that the best concentration was 250:1 (virus to formalin) and that the best temperature was 1° Celsius,
just a shade above the freezing point of water. Time
was a very critical factor. It was logical to assume that

the longer the virus was exposed to the formalin, the more virus would be killed. It was also correct to assume that the longer the exposure to formalin, the less antigenic the virus was likely to be.

After a batch of virus had been exposed to formalin, there remained the rather crucial problem of determining if any live virus remained. One way of doing this was to inject some of the hopefully dead virus directly into the brain of a monkey. If the monkey came down with polio, live virus was assumed to be in the batch. If the monkey did not sicken, it still could not be assumed that no live virus was in the batch; but if an injection directly into the brain did not bring the monkey down, then an intramuscular injection was even less likely to do so, and the batch was considered safe.

Just "safe" was not enough. The batch also had to be effective if it was to be any good as a vaccine. For a test of effectiveness, formalin-treated virus was injected intramuscularly, as it would be in humans, and the blood of the monkeys was tested for the presence and quantity of polio antibodies. However, results could never be certain. Monkeys are not people, the resemblance notwithstanding. One could never be certain that a batch of virus harmless to a monkey would not paralyze a human. There was always the possibility of a few live virus particles lying undetected in a given batch of vaccine. Nor did antibody formation in a monkey absolutely guarantee that the same injection would stimulate antibody production in a human. Batches were double-checked by seeing if they would grow in cultures of human cells. Failure to do so was a good indication of its safety, but by no means an infallible one.

Up to a point it was possible to detect live virus by injecting into monkeys, inoculating tissue cultures, challenging with immune serum, and other techniques. But beyond that point there was not enough live virus to give a positive test. Salk constructed a graph to record his observations. It consisted essentially of an ascending line that represented time and a descending line that represented detected virus. To obtain a margin of safety he extrapolated the graph by extending the exposure time as many days as possible beyond the point of no detectable virus before antigenicity was adversely affected. Assuming that the virus was killed at the same rate as observed on the graph, Salk was confident that all the virus could be killed without affecting the vaccine's antigenicity. Salk's critics argued that this was not a safe procedure because it assumed that the killing of the virus proceeded at the same rate regardless of the concentration of virus in the batch. Salk's assumption seemed reasonable enough, but when dealing with a material that was to be injected into children, "reasonable enough" was not enough, argued the critics.

By the spring of 1952 Salk and his staff were producing polio virus with factory-like efficiency. Monkeys injected with killed-virus stayed alive, with high blood antibody level, and successfully resisted challenge with live, virulent virus. In order to be injected, the virus had to be suspended in a liquid. Salk chose mineral oil, which served as an adjuvant—that is, it seemed to enhance the effect of the vaccine. The mineral oil held on to the virus at the injection site for a while before releasing it bit by bit. This probably acted somewhat as a repeating trigger for the body's anti-body-building mechanism, which resulted in more anti-body production than if the virus was released all at once. There was much disagreement over the use of adjuvants. Many thought they were too irritating and could even start cancers.

Salk was now at the stage where work with monkeys could tell him no more, and he felt the time had come for human testing. He could not proceed in this without the sanction and support of the foundation.

In 1952 the foundation's publicity mill saw to it that Bodian's finding of viremia was described on the front page of newspapers as an "encouraging development." This coincided nicely with the 1952 March of Dimes campaign, and although O'Connor received the usual angry letters from outraged scientists, the dimes poured in. It was indeed encouraging to the vaccine workers. The gamma-globulin trials had already shown that antibodies in the blood could prevent paralytic polio, and Bodian's work was additional evidence to help erase the doubts that vaccines might not work. Salk, Koprowski, and Sabin had shown that polio vaccines, dead or alive, injected or eaten, did raise blood antibody levels. Nobody knew just how much blood antibody was needed to be an effective block to polio virus, but the knowledge that polio virus entered the blood where antibodies could be ready and waiting to destroy them was encouraging.

The early 1950s was also a period of breakthrough for the biologist school of virology. These developments did not make the headlines but were the sort of thing the educated public could read about in *Scientific American* or, later, in the back pages of the *New York Times*. This work not only helped the immunologist school to understand better how viruses actually function, but it also led to a greater understanding of the molecular basis of heredity. These findings promise to have a far greater impact on the future of man than the polio vaccines.

In 1952 two American biochemists, A. D. Hershey and Martha Chase, clarified the mechanism of infection of bacteriophages, which are viruses that infect bacteria. The particular phage they investigated, called T-2, is a neighbor of polio virus, in that it inhabits the human intestine, which is normally replete with the bacterium *Escherichia coli*, the host cell of the T-2.

Bacteriophages were discovered in 1917 by Félix H. d'Hérelle, a Canadian-born bacteriologist, while he was working at the Pasteur Institute in Paris. He observed that certain bacteria were destroyed by what were first called "d'Hérelle bodies." After considerable controversy, it was determined that bacteriophages were indeed viruses, and that they somehow entered the bacterial cell and reorganized the substance of the bacteria to make more viruses. In many species, the bacterial cell spectacularly bursts to release thousands of new virus particles. Chemical analysis revealed that viruses, bacteriophages included, were made of an outer coat of protein and an inner core of nucleic acid, either DNA or RNA. Hershey and Chase determined that only the nucleic-acid core entered the bacteria. Since the naked nucleic acid alone was able to direct the reassembly of the substance of the bacteria into offspring viruses, it was then strongly suspected that nucleic acids were actually the hereditary material.

The work of Hershey and Chase stimulated others to determine the structure of DNA—among them, the American James D. Watson and the Englishman Francis Crick, who finally solved the problem in their work at Cambridge University in England. From that point on molecular genetics developed with mercurial rapidity. By 1962 it was understood how DNA actually directs the activities of cells; the genetic code was cracked. The bacteriophage came to be a most useful tool for molecular geneticists, and through work with this tadpole-shaped virus, actual genes were isolated and defined. The polio-vaccine work took place against the background of the molecular genetics explosion. Although it did not directly help the immunologists to make vaccines, it did eventually help them to understand why their vaccines work.

Regardless of how well a program goes in the laboratory, there remains the question of how a vaccine is to be tested. Using humans for testing has always been a bugaboo. From time to time proposals have been made to test preparations on institutionalized, mentally defective children or on convicts, and some projects have been carried out.

The foundation was fearful of such tactics for they could result in bad publicity, which was one of the reasons the foundation had been so annoyed with Koprowski for feeding of live virus to mentally defective children. This brought back memories of the Kolmer fiasco, which had followed the Brodie vaccine disaster. Kolmer had not been connected with the foundation in any way, but most people did not bother to make the distinction, and fund-raising drives had suffered following the deaths of children who had swallowed Kolmer's supposedly attenuated viruses. To many, it was too reminiscent of experiments done to children during the Nazi era.

Salk decided that a safe procedure would be to inject his vaccine into children who already had paralytic polio. These children were immune to whatever type of polio virus had caused their paralysis (determined by blood analysis), and an injection of a vaccine made of the same type virus could not do them any further harm. But if the vaccine was any good, the level of antibody in the blood would go up.

With the approval of the foundation, he made arrangements to test the vaccine at the Watson Home for Crippled Children in Leetsdale, Pennsylvania, a suburb of Pittsburgh. Many of the children there had had attacks of paralytic polio. Salk approached this phase of his work with caution and secrecy. He wanted no swarms of reporters disturbing him or the children. Foundation publicists did arrange to have pictures taken of the proceedings, but these were not released until a later time.

Some forty-five children were involved in the test. The initial step was to take blood samples so that the antibodies could be typed. Salk did this himself, then injected killed-virus that corresponded to the type of antibody the child possessed. He had taken every possible precaution, much more so than any of his competitors, but there was no way to eliminate all risk.

The injected children did indeed show a signifi-

cant rise in antibodies, and none of them showed the
vaguest symptom or any sign of illness. When at last he
injected vaccine into children with no previous history
of infection and no detectable antibodies, the results
were gratifying. The injected children developed a
high level of antibody and they all stayed healthy.

Salk did not subject the children to the danger of
injecting them with live virus in order to test the effectiveness of the vaccine. He took blood samples and introduced these into cell cultures of polio virus. The
cells continued to grow, an indication that the virus
had been destroyed.

There were no headlines. The work had been kept
secret, and Salk had maintained the anonymity and
therefore the privacy so important to a scientist who
wants to concentrate on his work. Soon after the results Salk informed Weaver and Rivers, but he did not
immediately publish them. He knew that the general
public did not read the journals but most science reporters did, and a story as newsworthy as this one
would soon have been in the daily papers.

However, the only way for Salk to find out if he
had a workable vaccine that was safe for general use
was to try it on a large number of people. Such an un-
dertaking could certainly not be kept secret. It would
require the cooperation of thousands of people, not the
least of whom were the virologist community. In a very
politic move, Weaver arranged to have the virologist
elite informed at a private meeting of the Immunization Committee in Hershey, Pennsylvania, on January
23, 1953.

Salk's report of the work with the Watson Home

children was received with great interest but with
mixed levels of enthusiasm. A virologist named Joseph
Smadel wanted to go right ahead with mass field testing. Sabin felt that even to talk about a field test was
premature and that years of preliminary work were
needed. He and others were concerned that the use of
virus grown in monkey kidney tissue might result in
damage to the recipient's kidneys. Enders tended to
side with Sabin. According to Rivers, Salk did not at
this time push for a field trial. Salk very carefully
avoided referring to his product as a vaccine; he called
it an "inactivated preparation."

The field-trial issue was not resolved at the Hershey meeting, and, in typical foundation style, it was
decided to expand the discussion at a larger meeting,
at which time the secrecy would certainly end. It was
January, March of Dimes time, and O'Connor was de-
lighted at the prospect of letting the world know of the
"tremendous progress" made by the young man in
Pittsburgh.

The big meeting convened in February of 1953 at
the Waldorf-Astoria Hotel in New York and was attended by such notables as the president of the American Medical Association (the AMA), the assistant surgeon-general of the United States, and deans and
professors from various prestigious medical schools.
Also included in this meeting, for some odd reason,
was the editor of the *Ladies' Home Journal*. Some of
the virologists in attendance were Salk, Rivers, Theiler,
and Smadel.

This was the first time that the progress of the vaccine work was made known to people outside the inner

circle of the foundation's virologist grantees. Those in attendance were brought up to date, then presented with the problems of field testing and informing the public. The decision was made to submit an article to the *Journal of the American Medical Association.*

The *Journal* is a professional medical publication more widely read by physicians than any of the more scholarly scientific journals. The cooperation of the medical community is very important in any such project. Doctors are understandably annoyed when accounts of some new medicine or medical technique are splashed all over the newspapers, and their patients, subsequently, begin to demand the new treatment. Publications such as the *Journal* give physicians at least a sporting chance to learn of new developments before everyone else in the country knows about them.

The proposed article was to present the progress so far made and caution against over-optimism and against a rush to inject the stuff into all available children. Because science editors of newspapers regularly read the *Journal,* the story would certainly find its way into the daily press. This would be the respectable route. It was also arranged for the *Journal* to run an editorial on the vaccine in the same issue. Field testing would commence as soon thereafter as possible.

This was a very good plan. It satisfied the foundation's need for publicity—beneficial to fund-raising—and the scientists' need to preserve professional integrity. However, the country did not learn of the vaccine from the AMA *Journal* and paraphrased newspaper articles but from a syndicated newspaper column called "Broadway," written by Earl Wilson. Wilson usually concerned himself with the activities and scandals of show-business personalities. It was just about the last place in the world one would expect to find news of science. The column was headed, "New Polio Vaccine—Big Hopes Seen."

Now everything that everybody did not want to happen happened. Parents started to demand the vaccine from their doctors, and virologists and other scientists chided Salk for being a publicity-seeker, which was one of the most devastating charges scientists could direct at a colleague. Salk, of course, had had nothing to do with the "leak" to Earl Wilson, and he was doubtless appalled at the prospect of losing esteem among his colleagues, many of whom were already beginning publicly to call him a "glory hound."

Salk went to New York to complain to O'Connor, and what followed can only be described as putting oil on the fire. It was arranged for Salk to make an address to the nation on a national radio and television network. This took place on the evening of March 26, 1953. It was a very good speech, in which Salk outlined the history of polio research and urged moderation and caution. Subsequently those scientists who had not been too sure about Salk's being a publicity-seeker were now convinced that he was. He had left the ivory tower and was now public property.

A newspaper story that appeared the following day left Salk with few supporters in the scientific fraternity. According to the story, the Parke Davis Company, one of the largest pharmaceutical companies in the country, would immediately begin to manufacture the vaccine. Many thought that Salk and/or the foundation had entered into some kind of deal with Parke Davis. Scientists and doctors were horrified at the thought that the vaccine would be put into use without testing. Actually the article was a piece of bad reporting; the story was just not true.

Parke Davis was, indeed, one of the companies that was to manufacture vaccine for the field trials. This same company had manufactured the adjuvant for the vaccine that Salk had used, but Salk himself had prepared the inactivated virus in his own laboratory. Suspicion ran strong because Salk was a paid consultant for the firm, although that in itself was not grounds for professional indictment, since many scientists served as consultants for a variety of industries and they were not drummed out of the scientific community for it. Furthermore, Parke Davis had previously suffered damage to its image from newspaper accounts of incidents involving one of its antibiotics, Chloromycetin. A number of deaths had occurred among recipients of this drug, but whether the deaths were due to any toxic qualities of the drug or to improper usage was not immediately clear.

Salk found himself in the middle of a tempest: the scientific world condemned him as a publicity hound; newspaper reporters and various foundation functionaries were annoyed with him and considered him an ingrate because he would not speak at fund-raising affairs. Money continued to flow into the foundation coffers from an anxious public, but Salk's standing within the scientific community had suffered damage that would linger for years.

O'Connor and the foundation publicity men saw in Salk the perfect hero, and they got all the mileage they could out of the hero concept, intentionally or not. Salk had all the qualifications: he was outwardly modest and self-effacing, young and reasonably good-looking, and had sprung from the New York tenements— the modern equivalent of the log cabin. Even his name had the ring of hero. It was short and terse, in the manner of Steve Canyon or Bobby Orr. (It is problematical if the foundation could have done as much with names such as Dorothy Horstmann or Hilary Koprowski.)

Now everybody knew, or at least wanted to believe, that the man in Pittsburgh had a vaccine that would save every mother's child from the evil virus of polio. Thanks to newspaper reports, people began to call it the Salk vaccine, and this made Salk uncomfortable. Smallpox vaccine was not called the Jenner vaccine, the yellow-fever vaccine was not called Theiler's vaccine, nor were the various bacterial disease vaccines referred to by the names of the men who developed them. Only Pasteur had been accorded such honor.

Salk was not even sure that he had a vaccine, in the precise sense of the word. In an attempt to ward off the embarrassment of appearing to seek after Pasteur-like sainthood, he referred to his material as the "Pittsburgh vaccine" or the "Pittsburgh preparation." But the word "Salk" was much more dramatic and more suitable for headline copy than "Pittsburgh" or even "Pitt.," which was also tried. "Salk vaccine" it has remained.

A
TIME
FOR
IMPATIENCE

CHAPTER VI

SALK CONTINUED HIS WORK AS WELL AS
he could, in the full knowledge that anything he did on
one day could be in the next day's newspapers. Reporters, like the Pittsburgh smog, were never far away.

All vaccine-makers are expected to administer
their product to themselves. This he did, and he also
injected the vaccine into his wife and three sons. About
500 more children in the Pittsburgh area were vaccinated without incident and with resultant rise in antibodies.

Spurred by Salk's work, O'Connor formed a new
committee, in early 1953, called the Vaccine Advisory
Committee, chaired by Rivers. The committee was to
get the vaccine tested and made available to the public
as soon as possible. By forming the committee,

O'Connor indicated that he was placing all his bets on Salk. O'Connor believed that he had a viable product in the Salk vaccine, even though he had been widely advised that an attenuated live-virus vaccine was probably better in principle than a killed-virus vaccine. Such vaccines were years away: the killed-virus vaccine was here and now. O'Connor was ready to commit all the foundation's resources and, indirectly, the integrity of his own name to promoting the Salk vaccine.

The new committee caused a great deal of resentment among the members of the old Immunization Committee. Most of the latter were not appointed to this committee. Hammon, Sabin, and Enders, to name just a few members of the Immunization Committee, were violently opposed in principle to killed-virus vaccines. Howard Howe, who was also a member of the Immunization Committee, still clung to fading hopes that his killed-virus vaccine would be the one elevated by the foundation. Only Joseph Smadel and Thomas Turner sat on both committees, and they were strong believers in killed-virus vaccines. Turner was a professor of bacteriology at Johns Hopkins and had worked with Bodian and Howe. Most of the new committee were public health people. O'Connor and Rivers explained the situation by saying that no one, including Salk, should be on the Vaccine Advisory Committee if he had any personal interest in any particular vaccine or other preventative. This explained the absence of Salk, Sabin, Hammon, and Howe, but not of Enders.

The Vaccine Advisory Committee met frequently in 1953 against a background of a growing fury over the vaccine. On the one hand there were local politicians and public health officials demanding vaccines for their districts in time for the next polio season; on the other hand there were those such as Sabin and Enders who insisted that the whole thing was a ghastly mistake. They were afraid of the Mahoney strain and skeptical of the safety of Salk's inactivation techniques. There was also professional jealousy, though scientists, who are supposed to be objective, would certainly deny that.

There was much furor in the meeting room itself, brought on by intense public pressure for a field trial in time for the 1954 polio season. There were many things to get together in a short time, ranging from pin-point specifications for the manufacturing pharmaceutical houses down to lollipops for the children.

Among the members of the committee there was agreement that the foundation should indeed run the field trials. However, there were several points of disagreement over how the trials were to be conducted. One was whether or not to use adjuvant, and the other was the matter of controls. One body of opinion favored injecting vaccine into one group and comparing the incidence of polio with an observed control group —that is, a group that received no injection of anything. Another favored the double blind control. The control group would receive an injection of a placebo such as saline solution (salt water), which would look like the real thing and, hopefully, sting like the real thing when injected. No one would know who was receiving which, not even the person giving the injection. The injections would be coded and the code

known only to an over-all administrator and his staff.
This was essentially the same double blind control that
had been used by Francis in the tests of his influenza
vaccine.

Those in favor of the double blind control argued
that this was the only way to avoid bias. Disease symptoms, including those of polio, are seldom as clear-cut
as described in the medical textbooks. A physician fa-
vorably disposed toward killed-virus vaccines might
tend to diagnose a heavy case of flu in the non-vacci-
nated control group as a mild case of polio. A doctor
who had no use for killed-virus vaccines might do the
same with a case of flu in the vaccine experimental
group. Those opposed to the use of a placebo agreed
that it added unnecessary risk. Some children could
become ill just from the injection itself. The observed
control proponents counseled that it was extremely un-
just to subject children to the risk and pain of an injection for nothing. They argued further that the presence
of a placebo in the trials would cause anxiety among
the parents, who would not know whether or not the
children they volunteered were protected.

The members of the committee did agree that an
over-all director of the field trials was needed. Joseph
Bell, a highly respected epidemiologist from the National Institutes of Health, was asked to do the job.
Bell immediately made it very clear to the committee
that he wanted a double blind control, with influenza
vaccine rather than saline solution as the placebo. The
committee thought this rather odd and gave him quite
an argument. Bell felt that the control group should

get some benefit out of participation, and as an epidemiologist he could not resist the prospect of the added
bonus of data on influenza vaccine.

Bell proposed a three-point safety check of the
vaccine. Each batch of vaccine would be tested in the
manufacturer's laboratory, Salk's laboratory, and in the
Laboratory of Biologics Control of the National Institutes of Health. This last was at Bell's strong insistence
and was the only involvement of any governmental
agency in the vaccine for the field trial. The foundation
was under no legal obligation to submit to governmental testing, and the contracted arrangement with the
National Institutes of Health was entirely voluntary on
the foundation's part.

Laws relative to the testing of medical products
were intended not to interfere with the progress of research in university or commercial laboratories. However, nothing approaching the magnitude of the proposed polio vaccine field trials had ever been attempted.
No one doubted that the foundation was sincere in its
efforts to eliminate polio, and the voluntary testing arrangement with the National Institutes of Health was
indicative of its sincerity. The foundation, despite its
size and quasi-official status, was nothing more than a
group of private citizens who now were taking it upon
themselves to arrange for the injection of a potentially
dangerous substance into hundreds of thousands of
children. It followed then that any group of citizens
could organize to inject anything into children, and as
long as parents volunteered their children, the group
would be within the law.

Salk was vigorously opposed to Bell's control recommendations, and he attended committee meetings to make his views known. This caused resentment among members of the Immunization Committee, such as Sabin and Howe, who had been barred from the Vaccine Advisory Committee on the grounds that no one with a personal interest in a vaccine could take part in its deliberations. Salk proposed that second-grade children in selected areas be injected with the vaccine, and that first- and third-grade children in the same areas serve as observed controls. The foundation people tended to favor Salk's plan, mainly because it was a simpler kind of field trial to run.

The vacillating members of the Vaccine Advisory Committee debated the issues of placebo *versus* observed controls, and of saline solution *versus* flu vaccine as the placebo, well into the fall of 1953, and with each day of bickering the possibility of organizing a field trial in time for the 1954 polio season became more remote.

While the committee argued, the foundation suffered two blows in quick succession in early fall of 1953. Harry Weaver resigned, mainly because he was not getting along with Hart Van Riper, the foundation's medical director. Weaver had accomplished more of the mechanics of getting the foundation as far as it was toward a vaccine and a field trial than any other one person. Having thorough knowledge of the basic essentials of research he had done whatever he felt had to be done to get the research going. Van Riper was primarily an administrator, without research experience, and his insistence on adhering to administrative protocol seemed like obstruction to Weaver.

Van Riper felt that Weaver was trying to run the whole show himself and was not keeping him informed about matters that the medical director should know, especially since, as medical director, Van Riper was supposedly in charge of the field trials. The Van Riper-Weaver conflict soon became a matter of "either he goes or I go," and Weaver was the one to go.

About the same time Bell resigned because he had become disgusted with the committee's deliberations, which each day became less discussion-like and more brawl-like. Bell did not need the foundation, they needed him; and if the foundation was not going to run the trials in a manner that he considered scientifically sound, then the trials would be run without him. He returned to the relative tranquillity of the National Institutes of Health.

So in October 1953 the foundation was replete with "withouts." It was without a director of research, and without an evaluator for a field trial that was without a plan—and with precious little vaccine. What it was not "without" was problems. Sabin continued to assail, publicly, the whole idea of a mass trial of a vaccine he described as unsafe.

One of the basic tenets of what is loosely referred to as the "scientific method" is the repeatability of experiments. Any researcher's conclusions are normally considered suspect until another researcher repeats the same procedure and achieves the same results. Repeating experiments has always been considered to be somewhat of a trial by peers among the scientific fraternity.

When Dr. Albert Milzer of the Michael Reese

Hospital tried to repeat Salk's work he kept getting live virus in the preparations. Van Riper insisted that Milzer surely had not followed Salk's methods exactly. Van Riper's public defense of Salk did nothing to improve Salk's image among his colleagues.

The pharmaceutical houses chosen to manufacture the vaccine were, in effect, large-scale repeaters of Salk's experiments, and they too were having difficulty producing the vaccine according to Salk's methods. Live virus was showing up in many batches of vaccine.

The companies insisted that they were following Salk's specifications and suggested to Salk that he make modifications.

Salk agreed to this, but weeks passed and he submitted no new specifications. The companies complained to Rivers and O'Connor, who pressured Salk. Salk was not procrastinating; he was having difficulty finding anything to change in his specifications. The inactivation process worked well in his laboratory, but something was obviously going wrong in adapting the process to large-scale production. Salk needed more time to investigate the problem, but there just was not any more time. O'Connor was getting frantic, and the requests for revised specifications became demands. The pharmaceutical houses had to start production if there was to be any field trial in 1954. Under pressure, Salk submitted essentially the same specifications as he had previously, but he described them in greater detail.

O'Connor had always taken pride in never interfering with foundation grantees, but the vaccine issue had now left the laboratory and was in the daily papers. There was much at stake. The pharmaceutical houses were getting impatient, and there existed the possibility that some of them might start making their own vaccine. Moreover Cox and Koprowski were making progress, and O'Connor lived in fear that any day they might announce that they were ready to start a field trial. The public wanted a vaccine in time for the 1954 polio season. If the vaccine was not ready, children might die who could have been saved.

The foundation had brought the public pressure on itself. For almost twenty years it had built up the image of polio as a national disaster. Summers were periods of dread. Every whimper, sniffle, vague muscle ache, and minor temperature increase in children terrorized parents. The fear had kept the money flowing; now the donors wanted results in return.

In 1953 the public had been told there was hope for a vaccine, although there would be none for that year. To be told now that there would be no field trial until 1955 would mean that no large-scale vaccinations would be available until 1956. The fear of polio, so skillfully promoted by the foundation's advertising, could trigger many reactions. As had been the case with gamma globulin, there would be desperate attempts to get what little vaccine was available. O'Connor could not repeat his tactic of buying up the entire supply. There was nothing to prevent pharmaceutical houses from utilizing the staff and know-how gathered from working with the Salk preparations to produce their own vaccine and test it in their own laboratories. They could then obtain a license to distrib-

ute it through normal commercial channels. There
were many in the country who would have liked that.
At some local and regional AMA meetings, resolutions
had been passed deploring the foundation's control of
the vaccine and the plans to give it away. Many of the
more conservative AMA members thought such plans
were nothing less than socialism, and they maintained
that the vaccine should be distributed according to the
traditional doctor-patient relationship of an office visit
followed by a bill. The Salk vaccine would require at
least three injections and, consequently, three office
visits.

By November 1953 it appeared that the Vaccine
Advisory Committee had argued itself out, and it announced that the field trial would be a double blind
study. Three days later O'Connor announced at a press
conference that the trials would be conducted with an
observed control. He stated further that the trials
would begin in February of 1954. It would seem that
Salk had made a final plea for an observed control, and
that O'Connor, Salk's champion, had had his way with
the committee.

A. Foard McGinnes, a public health physician and
an old friend of O'Connor, was put in charge of vaccine procurement. Six companies—Cutter, Eli Lilly,
Parke Davis, Pitman-Moore, Sharp & Dohme, and Wyeth
—were chosen to produce vaccine for the field trials.
However, vaccine from only two companies—Lilly
and Parke Davis—was actually used in the trials. When
O'Connor made his confident statement about a February starting date, the pharmaceutical companies were

still having trouble, and the only available vaccine was in Salk's laboratory, which was hardly equipped for mass production.

Despite the lack of vaccine, the Vaccine Advisory Committee assumed that there would indeed be a field trial, and after the decision was made on what kind of trial to run, consideration was given to the problem of evaluating it. As the idea of a field trial evolved after Salk's initial Watson Home trial, it was assumed that someone in the foundation would evaluate the trial. During Bell's short tenure he fell more or less into that role. After Bell left, re-examination of the problem resulted in the feeling that evaluation could not be haphazard and that in the interest of scientific objectivity the evaluator had best be someone not associated with the foundation.

The job of evaluator was offered to, and refused by, at least two people before thought was given to Salk's ex-teacher and mentor, Thomas Francis. Francis was on sabbatical leave in Europe, making a grand tour of various scientific meetings. Van Riper finally got a telephone call through to Francis in London. Francis made no commitment, but he said he would talk about it when he got back to New York in December.

Francis drove a very hard bargain. He would evaluate the field trial, but it would have to be done his way. He stated flatly that the trial would be a double blind study, and that is what it was. Not only did Francis overpower O'Connor on that issue, he also convinced Salk that that was the only way to do it. O'Connor was in somewhat of a bind. He had already

promised officials in several states that no placebo
would be used, therefore the tests in those areas would
have to be with observed controls. Conceding that
O'Connor had to keep his promise was the only point
on which Francis yielded. He realized that the limited
observed-control group could serve as a means of comparing the effectiveness of the two approaches.

Francis demanded that $900,000 be paid to the
University of Michigan and not to himself. All data
would be kept by Francis and his staff. No little tidbits
of "encouraging news" would be fed to O'Connor for
use in the March of Dimes mill. This last stipulation
was perhaps the hardest for O'Connor to take.

The Evaluation Center was set up at the University of Michigan, and by February, Francis was getting
things efficiently organized.

There was still no supply of vaccine. In January
1954 O'Connor had made a strategic retreat. He said
that, because of production problems, the start of the
trial would be delayed until March. That he was able
to say March 1954 and not March 1955, or even later,
was due to the relative success of Parke Davis and Eli
Lilly in producing safe vaccine. At least their record
was better than the other companies, but they still had
some problems.

Many people at the National Institutes of Health
thought that since some half a million children were
involved the government should be more directly concerned. The only governmental control was the contract that the foundation had voluntarily entered into
with the National Institutes of Health (NIH) for testing
batches of vaccine. The times were not conducive to

increased governmental control. President Eisenhower's choice for Secretary of Health, Education, and Welfare, of which the National Institutes of Health was a branch, was indicative of the administration's "don't make waves" attitude. Mrs. Oveta Culp Hobby, who had served as commander of the Women's Army Corps in World War II, was a charming, affable matron who served admirably as the token woman in the cabinet, but she was qualified neither in matters of health nor in education and welfare.

Concerned people in the National Institutes of Health could do little, but the little they could do proved to be bothersome to the foundation. The NIH insisted that merthiolate, an antiseptic, be added to the vaccine to kill any bacteria that might happen to be present. This annoyed Salk, who insisted that the antiseptic would spoil the effectiveness of the vaccine. The NIH said it would not pass the vaccine for use unless merthiolate was added.

In the early months of 1954 there was one crisis on top of another. Parke Davis reported that guinea pigs injected with one batch of vaccine showed a positive tuberculin reaction. The problem turned out to be a reaction to merthiolate rather than tuberculosis. The annoyance of this incident was compounded, since that particular batch was to be used to run tests in answer to critics who were afraid the vaccine would cause kidney damage. The necessity of clearing up the tuberculin mystery before the kidney safety tests could be started killed hopes of starting the field trial in March.

By March of 1954 some 7000 people, mostly children, had been given Salk vaccine without any adverse reaction. All the inoculated individuals demonstrated a rise in antibodies. Sabin continued to take every opportunity to speak out against the vaccine. Rather than attack Sabin directly, the foundation publicists arranged for Salk to speak to such groups as the American Academy of Pediatrics. Sabin was never mentioned in these speeches. Salk generally explained what had been done and what remained to be done.

In his speeches Salk admitted that the longevity of the immunity and the best way to space the injections were still unknown. On one point he and Sabin were diametrically opposed. Sabin maintained that the vaccine was actually harmful, because while the immunity lasted the body would not have a chance to build antibodies from natural exposure. Salk believed that the vaccine would trigger the body to keep on producing antibodies and was therefore as good as natural infection.

By March of 1954 Parke Davis and Lilly were finally producing vaccine in sufficient quantity for the field trial. A very stiff set of requirements had been drawn. Eleven consecutive batches of vaccine had to pass safety and potency tests in the producer's laboratory, Salk's laboratory, and in the National Institutes of Health laboratories before the vaccine could be released. There was a brief period of panic when some monkeys at the NIH laboratory collapsed after receiving some supposedly safe Parke Davis vaccine. Postmortem examination revealed that the monkeys did not have polio but some other virus disease quite common in monkeys.

As the nation had learned of Salk's initial successes

through a gossip columnist, so did it learn of the bad batches of vaccine. Walter Winchell, like Earl Wilson, was a syndicated columnist; he also had an evening news program, which was more sensation than news. His broadcasts always started with some piercing, simulated Morse signals followed by his staccato, "Good evening, Mr. and Mrs. America, and all the ships at sea." He would close his fifteen minutes of scandals, predictions, recriminations, and occasional praise (onions and orchids) "with lotions of love," an allusion to his hand-cream sponsor.

Winchell had no orchids or lotions of love for the foundation when he opened his April 4, 1954, broadcast with the words, "In a few moments I will report on a new polio vaccine—it may be a killer!" He went on to say, in his characteristic cryptic, dramatic style, that the United States Public Health Service had found live virus in ten batches of the vaccine. Winchell's informant was apparently Paul de Kruif, who had been out of the polio scene since the Brodie disaster.

The foundation responded with explanations that such tests were done routinely to eliminate the bad batches, which could be expected in any mass-production operation. Van Riper, at a press conference, went on to say that finding bad batches was actually a good thing, since it upheld the validity of the testing procedures.

A few localities dropped out of the trial. The foundation went ahead with plans to begin the trial in the last week of April 1954.

On April 24 the Vaccine Advisory Committee,

Salk, and Bodian met with NIH officials to decide whether or not to hold the field trial. The foundation people presented documents to the effect that over 7500 people had received the vaccine and there had been no kidney damage or other bad effects. They assured the NIH that the chosen pharmaceutical houses were producing potent, safe vaccine.

When the foundation people sat back to get the NIH scientists' "okay," they did not hear one. Rather, they heard a report that some mice had become paralyzed after inoculation with some batches of vaccine. Bodian replied with confidence that he knew the mice did not have polio. The mice, he contended, had died of something called Theiler's disease, a condition peculiar to mice and not men. Postmortems later corroborated Bodian's suspicion.

Bodian had never been too enthusiastic about killed-virus vaccines, and as a member of the Immunization Committee he had been bypassed in most of the important decisions involving the field trial. In an all too rare demonstration of the scientist's ostensible open-mindedness, he had not allowed personal feelings and jealousies to interfere with an objective judgment. If Bodian had so much as said "maybe" to the possibility of polio in the mice, the field trial might have been delayed to the point where it would have been too late for any trial at all in 1954.

The next morning the Vaccine Advisory Committee, with the blessing of the NIH, voted unanimously to start the field trial. The largest testing of a medical product in the history of man was about to begin.

THE
STING
OF THE
NEEDLE

CHAPTER VII ▄▄▄▄▄▄▄▄▄▄▄▄▄▄▄

Sᴛᴀʀᴛɪɴɢ ᴏɴ ᴍᴏɴᴅᴀʏ ᴍᴏʀɴɪɴɢ, April 26, 1954, children in the first, second, and third grades lined up in selected schools, armories, auditoriums, and gymnasiums to get stuck in the arm with a needle. No one at these proceedings knew whether any given child received a killed-virus vaccine or a placebo. (Both were pink liquids.) For their pains the children received, in most places, a lollipop. If they completed the series of three shots, they got a button with the words "Polio Pioneer" printed on it.

The test was divided into placebo areas and, thanks to O'Connor's politics, observed-control areas. When it was over, 441,131 children had received real vaccine, 201,229 had been injected with the placebo, and the 1,063,951 children who received nothing at all served as an observed control—that is, they were watched, as the others were, to see how many would get polio.

Nothing remotely like this had ever happened before. Tens of thousands of physicians, nurses, teachers, and other people volunteered their services. A union in a medical-equipment factory even stopped a strike so there would be enough hypodermic syringes and needles. The most remarkable volunteers were the parents. They volunteered their children with the full knowledge that some children would receive a placebo—in effect, an injection of nothing. They knew their children would be watched to see how many would become paralyzed or die, and they knew that some of the children would indeed become paralyzed and that some would surely die and become merely numerals on a computer read-out sheet.

The injections were finished in June, and while Francis and his group in Michigan gathered the data, O'Connor and the foundation gathered one crisis after another. Francis refused to look at any data until they were all collected. Evaluating the data was a much more complicated statistical exercise than just counting healthy, diseased, and dead children. Blood samples had to be taken from the participating children for antibody-level determination. Factors such as age, geographic location, and socio-economic status had to be fed into the calculations, in the proper statistical format. All of this took time. Francis would not give out any little bits of information no matter how persuasive the foundation publicists.

O'Connor had to make a decision whose magnitude made obtaining advance information a temptation that took the will of a saint to resist and made Francis's stubbornness hard to bear. O'Connor knew that if the field trial was successful there would have to be enough vaccine to meet the 1955 demand. To insure a sufficient supply, production would have to start before the results of the field trial were known. The pharmaceutical houses had tooled up for vaccine production and had hired high-priced personnel. They could not afford to let the equipment and people sit idle. Nor could they afford to produce vaccine that was not going to be licensed and therefore not used. The foundation had gotten them into the polio-vaccine difficulties and they now turned to the foundation for help.

O'Connor solved the problem with typical O'Connor dramatics. He promised to buy a total of $9,000,000 worth of vaccine from seven pharmaceutical houses. The vaccine would be dispensed free as far as it would go, with first choice to the children who had received placebo in the trial. Not a drop of it would be injected unless the results of the field trial were impressive enough to win a license from the Laboratory of Biologics Control. If no license was forthcoming, vaccine representing $9,000,000 of March of Dimes contributions would have to be poured down the nearest drain.

O'Connor's gesture implied that after this expenditure the foundation would go out of the vaccine business. Manufacturers would not have to pay any fees or royalties to the foundation, and the vaccine would be distributed through normal commercial channels. Vaccine might still be given away through local health agencies, but fee-conscious AMA members could no longer complain to the foundation.

In September 1954 practically every virologist and polio epidemiologist in the world was in Rome to attend the Third International Poliomyelitis Conference. The atmosphere was more like that of the court of the Borgias in Renaissance Florence than a scientific conference. Little effort was made to conceal the animosity between the live-virus and the killed-virus schools, and there were washroom intrigue and smoke-filled-room maneuvering. Scientific objectivity was only a textbook phrase as supporters of Sabin or Salk nurtured hopes of deposing the leader of the opposite school.

Dr. Sven Gard, a noted Swedish virologist and a Sabin supporter, reported that Salk's inactivation graph was not a straight line representing a steady rate of virus kill but a diminishing curve with a decreasing rate of kill. Gard maintained that antigenicity was destroyed before all the virus was killed and that the vaccine, therefore, could not possibly be both safe and effective. His vehement defense of his conclusions seemed a little after the fact. By that time almost 450,000 human beings had received Salk's preparation, a massive polio epidemic had not broken out, and post-injection increases in antibody levels had been demonstrated.

Salk, Sabin, Koprowski, and their followers spoke in turn, each defending his position and taking every opportunity to try to destroy the opposition. There was little of the compromise and mutual exchange that were supposed to occur at scientific meetings. Minds were closed: there was only attack and parry. An effort intended for the "good of mankind" had brought science to a low point.

Meanwhile, in the United States, there was more trouble for Salk and the foundation. Routine testing of stored, commercially produced vaccine revealed that many batches had lost potency. There had been no such problem with the field trial since the vaccine had been used quickly; indeed, most of it had been produced barely in time for use in the trial.

The vaccine involved in the potency-loss problem was that which O'Connor and the foundation had underwritten. The problem was quite serious since in the normal course of commerce the vaccine would have to be stored. The difficulty was found to be the merthiolate, which had destroyed much of the antigenicity of the vaccine. The foundation requested permission from the National Institutes of Health to stop putting merthiolate in the vaccines. The NIH replied that a merthiolate-less vaccine could not be licensed unless a new field trial was conducted. Rivers was, in his own words, "sore as hell" at the NIH position. The NIH had insisted on the merthiolate in the first place.

Rivers and the Vaccine Advisory Committee did not retreat this time. They knew that the removal of the merthiolate would in no way affect the safety of the vaccine, and they were not about to go to the expense of another field trial. A compromise was worked out whereby 5000 to 8000 children would be inoculated with vaccine that had no merthiolate, to obtain clinical evidence that it was safe and effective.

Through the late summer, fall, and winter of 1954 various newspapers attempted to take straw polls of people involved in the field trial in an effort to get some advance information. For the most part the various health officials kept their word to Francis and told the reporters nothing. No one person could have provided any meaningful information in any case. Articles predicting the outcome appeared in newspapers, various magazines, Sunday supplements; writers related information from "reliable sources." It was almost like a summer before a political convention. The incidence of polio did go down in 1954, but there had been low incidence in other years, so no conclusions could be made from case totals. At least it was known that the vaccine itself had not caused an epidemic.

O'Connor waited anxiously for Francis to prepare his report. Francis said it could not possibly be ready before the end of 1954, indicating that March 1955 was a likely date. There would, in that case, be another frantic rush. The vaccine would have to be licensed before it could be used for the 1955 polio season, and March was almost too late to get a program going. There was the possibility that the NIH people might debate the licensing issue for months, and then there would surely be no vaccination program for the 1955 polio season.

Francis had his report ready by April 1955, and the manner chosen to disclose the report was in curious contrast to the model of scientific objectivity that had been Francis's evaluation.

The usual manner of reporting any scientific endeavor was to submit an article to a journal or to read a paper on the work at some conference of appropriate scientists. The foundation people were afraid that traditional methods would take too long and not have the proper effect to bring about a fast licensing. That consideration perhaps explains why Francis agreed to the circus that took place on April 12, 1955.

Arrangements were made for Francis to read the report at the University of Michigan in Ann Arbor. Attendance would be by invitation and the audience composed of notables in virology, medicine, public health, and other fields of science. The proceedings were to be telecast via closed circuit to doctors gathered in selected movie theaters throughout the country. The closed-circuit telecast was paid for by the Eli Lilly Company, which was only one of the companies producing the vaccine.

John Enders did not attend the proceedings at Ann Arbor. He offered excuses but it was clear that he wanted no part of it.

April 12 was the anniversary of the death of Franklin D. Roosevelt, and the choice of this date seemed to imply that it had been chosen for dramatic effect. The foundation spokesmen explained that April 12 was the earliest feasible date and that no dramatics were intended. Rivers made no excuses. He blustered that FDR had started the whole thing and to honor him in connection with the vaccine was an appropriate thing to do.

The reading of the report was carried off with more dignity than could be expected in a hall jammed with television and newsreel cameras, floodlights, and cables. But there was no dignity in the pressroom. Arrangements had been made to distribute copies of Francis's evaluation to about 150 reporters one hour before Francis was due to speak. The reporters had agreed to instruct their newspapers, radio and television stations not to release the news until 10:20 A.M. when Francis was scheduled to begin.

When university employees bearing copies of the report walked into the pressroom, the reporters descended upon them in a body. To the messenger boys, the mass of reporters must have appeared as a single amoebalike monster with hundreds of outstretched, grasping arms. The messengers panicked and threw their copies at the reporters, who scrambled and fought for them.

Francis delivered his report in a monotone, with very few superlatives or even adjectives. Those in attendance knew they were listening to a classic of objective scientific evaluation. When he got to the actual results of the trial, which was what everyone was waiting for, they turned out to be mixed. The vaccine was judged to be about 60 to 70 per cent effective against Type I polio virus and over 90 per cent effective against Types II and III. The incomplete effectiveness against Type I was unfortunate since it was the most frequent cause of paralytic polio.

Francis was able to show that the vaccine was about 94 per cent effective in preventing bulbarspinal paralysis, a severe form of polio that results in respiratory paralysis and, frequently, death. The vaccine was not at all effective against the mild intestinal form of the disease, and that was encouraging. A natural intestinal infection was still recognized as the most effective

way to immunization. This was effective evidence to
refute Sabin's contention that the killed-virus vaccine
would prevent the acquisition of natural immunity.
Even if the immunity conferred by Salk's vaccine was
indeed temporary, the recipient could possibly develop
natural immunity while the temporary immunity lasted.

The news reached much of the American public
before Francis began talking. Dave Garroway of the
National Broadcasting Company could not resist
making the announcement on his morning program
about 9:30, in violation of the unofficial agreement. So,
just as Francis started to read the report, church bells
were ringing and sirens sounding. Principals of schools
came through on public-address systems, calling for
moments of silence in thanks to Dr. Salk. The same
thing occurred in factories and offices. Hastily written
Thank you, Dr. Salk signs appeared in and on store
windows. Men and women openly wept on the streets,
and special prayer meetings were called in churches
and synagogues.

There had never been such a massive outpouring
of emotion over a medical product. Diphtheria and typhoid fever had killed many more thousands of children than had polio, but church bells had not greeted
the control of these diseases. Much of the national reaction was due to the foundation's publicists, who had
built up the image of polio as a massive plague. The
cries of thanks were not directed at the foundation and
at Basil O'Connor but at Jonas Salk. The 1950s were
bland times; the level of public excitement was geared
to news of the "cold war" or the convictions of such figures as Alger Hiss and the Rosenbergs, with the sordid

hysteria of the McCarthy hearings as an underlying theme. People were weary of looking in closets for lurking Communists. They wanted a hero, and now they had one in Salk.

When Francis finished speaking there was moderate applause. Salk spoke next. It was a speech that annoyed Rivers and many of the other scientists at the meeting. The source of the annoyance was Salk's statement to the effect that if it had been possible to give the third shot seven months after the second, as he had recommended, there would have been greater effectiveness in the results of the trial. He went on to talk about the merthiolate problem, and, to many, seemed to imply that Francis should have calculated the results of the merthiolate vaccine separately from the non-merthiolate vaccine. This implied criticism of Francis angered many, and Salk's opening words of praise for Francis did nothing to allay the anger. Salk ended his talk by saying that the new 1955 vaccine, used according to his procedures, could theoretically be 100 per cent effective. That last statement made the cautious Francis quite angry. No vaccine had ever been 100 per cent effective.

There was still the matter of licensing the vaccine, which usually required months of examination, re-evaluation, and discussion. Since nothing else about the vaccine had been usual, there was no reason to expect that licensing would follow precedent. Mrs. Hobby and Surgeon-General Leonard A. Scheele were waiting in Washington in front of reporters and television and newsreel cameras. Mrs. Hobby had had nothing to say about the vaccine during the previous hectic two years, and no one expected her to say anything now. Nonetheless she was, by the grace of the President and the Senate of the United States, the Secretary of Health, Education, and Welfare, and the vaccine could not be distributed until she signed the licensing document.

An open telephone line was maintained between Mrs. Hobby and a committee assembled in an Ann Arbor hotel. The committee consisted of some fifteen virologists gathered by William Workmann of the Laboratory of Biologics Control of the National Institutes of Health. Included were Sabin, Salk, Hammon, Smadel, and Bodian. Enders, as has been mentioned, had been invited but had chosen not to appear. This committee was to examine the report and make recommendations to Workmann, who would relay them to Scheele, who was delegated to tell Mrs. Hobby that it was all right to sign the license.

A man standing trial does not buy champagne to celebrate his acquittal while the jury is still out, but the open phone line with Mrs. Hobby waiting in front of the mass media, had been set up even as Francis was delivering the report. The entire nation seemed to be waiting with rolled-up sleeves for the deliverance from polio. It was April, and the polio season had already started in the southern states. Workmann did not actually tell the committee to hurry, but it was clear that the committee had best not take too long to go through Francis's fifty-page report, the book-length production records from the pharmaceutical companies, and the records of the Laboratory of Biologics Control tests. It is perhaps remarkable that the committee was able to keep Mrs. Hobby and O'Connor waiting for as long as two hours, but that was how long they deliberated.

All the old questions were brought up—the Mahoney strain, the high incidence of batches with live virus, and the reliability of testing procedures. Many on the committee, notably Sabin, wanted more time, but everyone knew that there was no more time. Workmann announced that each batch would be approved on the basis of the protocols of the manufacturer —that is, the production records. His laboratory would not retest the batches. That would be time-consuming, Workmann said, and the Laboratory of Biologics Control was not set up for such large-scale testing.

The committee unanimously recommended licensing. A smiling Mrs. Hobby signed the licensing papers while the cameras were trained and the flash bulbs popped.

In the weeks that followed, the honors and proposed honors that rained upon the balding head of Jonas Salk ranged from the pompous to the ridiculous. Some Texans wanted to give him some farm machinery and an automobile. Salk suggested that they be sold and the money used to buy vaccine. A congressman proposed, on the floor of Congress, that a Jonas Salk dime be struck. Designs for this were actually submitted. Magazines badgered him for exclusive stories, and several Hollywood movie studios wanted to do his life story. President Eisenhower invited him to the White House to receive a special presidential citation.

An adoring public was ready to give Salk anything, including a pension of $10,000 a year for life, suggested by another congressman. Salk knew better than to accept any money for personal use. Even that rejected offer backfired into more disapproval from the scientific community. Many newspapers editorialized on how wonderful it was that Salk had refused royalties or other payment for his "discovery." But Salk had not "discovered" anything—and even though he had never remotely entertained thoughts of remuneration, repeated referrals to his "noble attitude" further angered scientists. What Salk wanted and needed— honors from the scientific community—did not come to him. However, Mount Sinai Hospital, where he had not been offered a position after his internship, did give him a citation.

In 1954, as has been mentioned, Enders, Weller, and Robbins received a Nobel Prize for their polio virus tissue-culture work. Salk had been discussed as a candidate at Nobel Committee meetings, but the necessary recommendation of other virologists was just not forthcoming. One of the members of the Karolinska Institutet of Stockholm, where Nobel winners are determined, was the same Sven Gard who had denounced Salk's vaccine as unsafe if effective and ineffective if safe.

Very few scientists win Nobel Prizes, and so time expended in lamenting over prizes not won is not considered to be time well spent. However, many scientists who have done original work belong to the National Academy of Sciences, the most prestigious body of scientists in America. Membership is an accolade earnestly sought after by most research scientists. Salk was not admitted. The ostensible reason was that Salk had not done any *original* work—he was neither the first nor the only researcher to have prepared a for-malin-inactivated vaccine. The real reasons for refusal were the press conferences, radio and TV appearances, the *Life* magazine spreads, the mad scenes at Ann Arbor, Salk's alleged slurs at Francis, the outpouring of public adoration, and all the other violations of the sci-entists' unofficial code of behavior.

Although pharmaceutical stocks rose after the re-port at Ann Arbor, the advance was temporary and the companies chosen to manufacture the vaccine found little cause for rejoicing. They were having as much trouble with the 1955 vaccine as there had been with the field-trial batches. Many batches of vaccine had to be thrown away because of live virus. This was very expensive and was eating away the profits. The com-panies did not publicize their problems. They were re-quired only to submit protocols on batches to be re-leased, and the bad batches were quietly disposed of.

The vaccination program went reasonably well in the weeks following Ann Arbor. There was not as much vaccine available as had been hoped for, but there never had been enough, and that was accepted as an inconvenience that could be corrected as the pro-gram continued.

When a case of paralytic polio occurred in a vacci-nated one-year-old child in Chicago on April 24, 1955, no one was particularly alarmed. The child had re-ceived the first shot only ten days before, and it was as-sumed that the disease had been incubating before the shot was given. This had happened in a few instances during the field trial, and it was expected to occur again. It did.

On April 26 Robert Dyer of the California Health Department called the National Institutes of Health to report that six vaccinated children in California had come down with paralytic polio a week to ten days after receiving their first shot. There were two observations that made this report hair-raising rather than routine. All the children were paralyzed in the arm that received the vaccine, and in every case the vaccine had been prepared by the Cutter Company. Polio paralysis usually occurred in the legs. The six-in-a-row incidence of arm paralysis was not only suspicious, it was chillingly reminiscent of the Brodie disaster of 1935.

James Shannon, the assistant director of the NIH, quickly called a meeting of NIH officials. It convened at 7:30 P.M. on April 26 and went on until almost 5:00 A.M. the next day. The eight men at the meeting could not agree whether or not the events in California clearly indicated that something was wrong with the Cutter vaccine. There were only three clear choices: continue the program as it was; continue but take the Cutter vaccine off the market; suspend the entire program.

Surgeon-General Scheele was brought into the discussion by telephone at 3:00 A.M. It is not clear just what the NIH men expected him to do for them at three o'clock in the morning. Some decisions obviously had to be made immediately, but even the head of public medicine in the country could not be expected to make such awesome decisions when he was not fully awake.

There was nothing good about any of the choices. If the program was continued and the vaccine was indeed bad, the worst polio epidemic in history might occur. Cutter's problems just might have been repeated in other companies, and the withdrawal of the Cutter product, only to have the same thing happen with another company's vaccine, could cause nationwide hysteria. Suspending the entire program would destroy public confidence and possibly result in an increased incidence of polio. Even in his sleepy state Scheele must have known that the decision was his alone to make, which he was not willing to do at that hour. He suggested that virologists such as Rivers, Francis, Sabin, and Salk be contacted.

The first consultations with the virologists were by conference telephone calls early in the morning of April 27. If Scheele expected a unanimous recommendation from these men he was thinking wishfully. Disagreement among scientific colleagues was a way of life. The expert opinions ranged from continuation of the program to immediate suspension. The only point of agreement was that they would all go along with whatever the Surgeon-General decided to do.

Less than eight hours after he had heard of the events in California, Scheele made his decision to get the Cutter vaccine off the market and to continue the program with the vaccine produced by other pharmaceutical houses. Actually the Surgeon-General had no authority arbitrarily to order the Cutter vaccine off the market. He sent a telegram to Cutter, requesting that the company stop distributing the vaccine, and the president of the Cutter Company did so immediately. Within thirty minutes the message had been relayed to all Cutter distribution offices.

The withdrawal of the Cutter vaccine was one of the fastest governmental decisions in the history of the United States. It took almost three times as long to declare war on Japan following the attack on Pearl Harbor. The decision to take some vaccine off the market took four times as long as the time spent in deliberating the licensing of the vaccine. The same virologists who, unanimously, though hastily and under pressure, had advised Scheele to give a favorable judgment to Mrs. Hobby on the licensing would probably have debated the Cutter issue for two years and still not been able to offer a unanimous recommendation.

The Executive Branch of the United States Government had largely stood by and watched while the foundation had its way with 400,000 children in the field trial. By April 1955 some 5,000,000 children had received commercial vaccine. Scheele, as a part of the Executive Branch, had to make public statements to an anxious and frightened populace. The California polio cases and the withdrawal of the Cutter vaccine certainly could not be kept secret, and although Scheele had been forceful in his decision-making he could not quite bring himself to be completely honest with the press. He tried to pass off the Cutter withdrawal as a "safety precaution" and assured the reporters that there was no cause for alarm. The vaccination program, he told them, would continue.

But there *was* cause for alarm, and neither the reporters nor most of the public were fooled by Scheele's platitudes. Doctors advised their patients not to take Salk vaccine, at least until the situation was clarified. Meanwhile there were more vaccine-associated cases of polio. Twenty-two cases occurred in vaccinated children in Idaho; all had taken Cutter vaccine. Public health people really began to get scared when the disease spread to people who had been in contact with the vaccinated victims. There existed the grotesque possibility of the first vaccine-induced epidemic. Emergency supplies of gamma globulin were gathered.

There was no epidemic, but there were about 250 vaccine-associated cases, including the contacts. About 150 of the cases involved complete or partial paralysis, and there were 11 deaths. When compared to the 5,-000,000 people who had received the vaccine, the 250 Cutter cases and another 115 cases among vaccinated children seemed like a very good record for the vaccine. Another 130 cases of polio were probably coincidental. These beautiful statistics were no comfort to the parents of the stricken children, or to Salk, the foundation, or the Cutter Company.

Few people attempted to identify Salk as the villain, but he was no longer quite the hero figure he had been one month earlier. Nor was the foundation really the heavy, although O'Connor angered many people when he publicly disclaimed any responsibility on the part of the foundation. The medical profession in general was annoyed at the foundation for fostering the rapid licensing of the vaccine. Once it had been licensed, the physicians could not refuse the demands of their patients for the vaccine.

The Cutter Company, as a commercial enterprise, was a natural target of public wrath. The public felt that the company's rush for profit had killed little children. In fact, the Cutter Company had carefully followed procedures, and their employees and the employees' children had taken the vaccine. It does not seem likely that anyone would permit his children to be injected with a substance he even suspected of being shoddily made. With the removal of the Cutter vaccine, the number of vaccine-induced cases declined, and by June 1955 there were no more.

What was really frightening about the Cutter incident was not so much the number of cases but the fact that it had happened. The thought was always present that if it had happened to Cutter, a highly respected pharmaceutical house, it could happen to any of the other companies involved, all of whom were having trouble with live viruses in the vaccine.

The others were luckier. They detected the bad batches, and vaccine containing live virus never left the confines of their laboratories. That something was wrong, however, was obvious, and luck could not be tolerated as even an unofficial part of a vaccine-producer's protocols. What had happened and how it had happened had to be determined.

Starting immediately after the Cutter vaccine was stopped, there were many meetings. All the eminent figures in virology were involved in these meetings, which ranged from secret conclaves to congressional hearings.

Preliminary examination of the Cutter plant and the company's records revealed nothing out of order, and that was disturbing. The investigators would have been very happy to find some deficiency at Cutter, but the strict adherence to the Salk procedure that they found there increased the fear that bad vaccine pro-

duced elsewhere could again find its way into the arms
of children.

Immediately under fire were Salk's inactivation
curve and the Mahoney strain. A prevalent opinion
among the virologists was that Salk's safety margin in
the exposure time to formalin was not long enough, especially in reference to the Mahoney strain. Many virologists thought the Mahoney strain was too difficult
to kill to be safely used in a vaccine, and when John
Enders recommended that the entire vaccination program be stopped until the Mahoney-strain problem
could be investigated further, Scheele did as Enders
recommended. The program was stopped on May 7,
and Scheele uttered more banalities to the press and to
the public in a television appearance on May 8. He
said, then, that the action should not be interpreted as
implying that anything was wrong with the vaccine.
But it was difficult for the reporters and the public to
believe that nothing was wrong with the vaccine if the
vaccination program was being stopped. In the televised statement Scheele reminded everyone that the
number of polio victims was very small compared to
the 5,000,000 vaccinations. He said that the suspension
of the program was being made in order to allow time
for a double check of all the vaccine manufacturers. He
closed his remarks with praise for Salk and the foundation.

Salk was crushed, O'Connor furious, and congress-
men made outraged statements on the slipshod way
the vaccine had been inspected. Actually there had
been no inspection at all. The National Institutes of
Health had examined only the production records that

the manufacturers had chosen to release. The NIH had not inspected any post-trial vaccine, and it knew nothing of the manufacturers' problems in keeping live virus out of the vaccine. The pharmaceutical houses were examined, and a week after Scheele's announcement some Lilly vaccine was released, paving the way for a slow resumption of the vaccination program. There were few takers, for public confidence had been shaken.

A few companies reported they were still having trouble. Some of the virologists who had been consulted were organized into an *ad hoc* technical committee. One of its first recommendations was that the manufacturers be required to inform the NIH of any bad batches.

On May 23 Dr. Louis Gebhardt of the University of Utah actually detected live Mahoney Type I virus in a sample of Cutter vaccine. Until that time all action had been taken only on the assumption that live virus was in the vaccine. The Gebhardt work confirmed the suspicions of those committee members who believed the Mahoney strain to be the root of the problem. That same day the committee met at the NIH to consider tighter specifications for the manufacturers. The pharmaceutical houses complained about the added expense but went along.

Some of Scheele's public statements were unfortunate, and although his actions were open to criticism it is problematical whether any of his critics would have handled the Cutter incident in any other way. The vaccine affair had forced him into a "damned if you do, damned if you don't" situation. His biggest mistake was allowing himself to be pressured into licensing the vaccine only two hours after the Francis report. But had he insisted on a longer examination period, he would have been cast as the villain who was deliberately keeping life-saving vaccine from children. Mrs. Hobby's greatest contribution was a statement that has become a classic in the history of incredible statements made by public officials. At a press conference she said, "No one could have foreseen the public demand for the vaccine."

In June 1955 Scheele dutifully submitted a 162-page report on the Cutter incident to Mrs. Hobby. In the report he took issue with the Salk inactivation graph; criticized the Laboratory of Biologics Control for examining production records rather than actual vaccine; and implied criticism of the foundation for encouraging the rushed licensing procedure. Even if Mrs. Hobby were capable of doing anything about the problems described in the report, she never gave herself the chance. She resigned in July.

That month many of the leading virologists had a chance to make known their views when Representative Percy Priest called a hearing before the House Committee on Interstate and Foreign Commerce. This committee was considering a bill to appropriate $25,-000,000 to buy vaccine for children of low-income families.

Sabin was there, and, as expected, he spoke against the vaccine. He said that the vaccine was not consistently safe; that anyone who took the vaccine was a potential sacrificial lamb for others who might be protected by it. Previously, at an AMA symposium,

Sabin had made it known that he was making progress on his own attenuated strains for a live-virus vaccine.

Wendell Stanley expressed the opinion that the course of the reaction between formalin and virus was impossible to predict because of the varying nature of viruses. He said that there could be undetected viable virus in any batch of vaccine. Salk countered by claiming that there was a "point of no return" in the formalin reaction beyond which no virus could return to a living state.

Rivers took up Salk's cause, trading verbal blows with Stanley and Sabin. He picked up Sabin's admission that the Salk vaccine was safe, at least most of the time, to chide Sabin for suggesting that a safe vaccine be denied to those who might benefit from it until he could make a better one. He reminded Stanley that formalin was an "old friend" of vaccine workers, and he challenged Stanley to suggest a better way of inactivating viruses.

Rivers' support of Salk was very significant. He was one of the most respected virologists in the country, and it had been his opposition to the Brodie and Kolmer vaccines that had stopped the use of those preparations. Had he not supported Salk, it is possible that the inactivated-vaccine program would have been discontinued permanently.

Enders stated that he agreed with Sabin and came out very strongly in favor of discontinuing the Mahoney strain.

Francis agreed with Enders on the Mahoney strain, but he stated that an attenuated vaccine could possibly have active virus in it too, and that such vaccines would have no monopoly on safety.

As long as they were together, it was agreed to take an unofficial vote on two questions, the Mahoney strain and the continuance of the program. There was tacit agreement that how they voted was the way the Salk vaccine would go. Salk abstained from the voting; Stanley and Manfred Mayer of Johns Hopkins also abstained, on the grounds that they were not physicians. The vote to remove the Mahoney strain was unanimous. The vote was eight to five in favor of continuing the program. Among the negative votes were those of Sabin and Enders. Hammon had indicated in a letter to Sabin that he was opposed to continuing the Salk program.

The reason for the Cutter incident was never clearly established. The technical committee did offer a probable cause. Bottles of tissue-culture fluid containing the virus had been stored before going through the formalin-inactivation process. Bits of tissue-culture debris had then settled to the bottom and covered virus particles, protecting them from the formalin. The committee recommended that the tissue-culture fluid be filtered to remove the debris before exposure to formalin.

The problem had not occurred during the field trial since vaccine was produced so fast that the bottles of tissue-culture fluid did not have a chance to stand long enough for much settling to take place. The explanation seemed to fit, since vaccine produced by Salk in his own laboratory had never caused paralysis.

Most of the men who had been involved in the

two-hour licensing deliberation had had experience with growing virus in tissue culture, but as far as is known the possibility of virus getting trapped in bits of tissue was not discussed there. The pressures of a waiting nation had precluded much discussion at that meeting, and, after all, Salk had assured reporters at Ann Arbor that "the vaccine is safe, and you can't get safer than safe."

SYRUP
AND
SUGAR
CUBES

CHAPTER VIII ▰▰▰▰▰▰▰▰▰▰▰▰▰▰▰▰

IN 1946 POLIO RESEARCH WAS STILL in the dark ages. The Johns Hopkins group and John Enders had yet to inform the world that there was more than one type of polio virus, that the polio virus was not exclusively neurotropic, and that polio virus would grow in practically any kind of living cell. Most virologists still doubted the possibility of a safe polio vaccine. Yet that year the Lederle Division of the American Cyanamid Company decided to commit itself to developing a live-virus polio vaccine.

The venture was initiated with enthusiasm and confidence. Much of the optimism was directly traceable to Hilary Koprowski and Herald Cox, who assured Lederle that the vaccine could be made and that the company would be richer and more famous for the effort. That a commercial enterprise was willing to invest millions in what was essentially a basic research problem was amazing. That they kept it up as long as they did was even more amazing.

While Salk was developing his killed-virus vaccine, he and the foundation considered Cox and Koprowski their strongest competitors. Much of the urgency and speed of the foundation's vaccine efforts stemmed from the fear that Lederle would be first, stealing the foundation's thunder. The whole concept of voluntary organizations such as the foundation would have been undermined by a successful Lederle effort.

There was good reason to believe that Cox and Koprowski would make the first successful polio vaccine. Between them they had a long history of vaccine successes for other diseases. They had at their disposal the vast financial resources of Lederle, recently made much vaster by the success of Aureomycin, an antibiotic developed at Lederle.

Pharmaceutical companies, like other commercial enterprises, are seldom in a position to invest millions of dollars in basic research programs that may or may not result in black ink on the ledger book. The usual procedure has been to rely on promising basic research done in a university or institute laboratory. This research is then expanded to devise medications with the greatest therapeutic effect and least toxicity or side effects at the greatest possible profit.

Cox and Koprowski had previously developed for Lederle a rabies vaccine that was a great improvement over Pasteur's, and it was very profitable. The virus was grown in duck eggs rather than in rabbit spinal cords. Before coming to Lederle, Cox had been with the United States Public Health Service. He had worked with rickettsiae, those strange organisms that seem to be intermediate between viruses and bacteria. He had devised techniques for culturing rickettsiae in avian eggs and had developed vaccines against two rickettsial diseases, typhus and Rocky Mountain spotted fever. He had also helped to isolate the virus that causes a disease called Q fever. He came to Lederle in 1942 and developed many successful veterinary vaccines for preventing diseases of hogs, dogs, and chickens. In 1944 he invited Koprowski to join him at Lederle.

Koprowski was a living refutation of the common belief that scientists are of necessity a narrow and boorish lot of people who know nothing outside their own specific fields. He was a graduate of Warsaw Medical School and the Warsaw Conservatory of Music. In addition to being an accomplished pianist, he was a linguist and could converse brilliantly in any number of fields. Frequently he embarrassed his less literary colleagues with allusions to mythology and literature in his papers and presentations. Ostensibly working under Cox, Koprowski actually ran the Lederle vaccine project.

Lederle certainly seemed to have a winning team, but with all of Cox's experience, Koprowski's urbanity and skill, and Lederle's bags of money, they made the same mistake as had Brodie and Kolmer. They were working with the old ideas of polio. As the orthodoxies were overthrown by Morgan, Bodian, Howe, and Enders, the troubles at Lederle got bigger.

Cox and Koprowski started their work by passing a virus, known as the TN strain, through cotton rats. This virus had been extracted from a human subject. Virus was recovered from the rats, injected into other rats, recovered and injected into still others, and so on. This was essentially the same procedure used by Pasteur to attenuate rabies virus. Cox and Koprowski tested the virus for attenuation by injecting it directly into the spinal cords of monkeys. The rationale here was that if virus so drastically administered to a monkey failed to bring the animal down, then the same virus was not likely to harm a human being who swallowed it. The monkey test was crude, but it was all they had. (Enders had not yet shown the virologists that tissue cultures could be used to test for virus activity.) The monkey test could not tell them whether or not the virus was over-attenuated and therefore ineffective for use in a vaccine. The only way to test this was to feed the virus to an appropriate animal and then check the recipient's blood for antibodies. They first tried feeding their attenuated virus to chimpanzees, which survived and showed antibodies. By January 1950 they felt they were ready to follow tradition and take their own vaccine. They did so, suffered no ill effects, and in later tests discovered antibodies in their own blood. They were the first people willingly to swallow live polio virus, with no resulting sickness, and to receive the added bonus of developing antibodies.

Salk, still typing viruses, had not even submitted a vaccine proposal. Salk was only a name, not a threat, but the typing project that Salk and others were carrying out was a threat. By 1950 there was no doubt that

there were at least three types of polio virus. Cox and
Koprowski had spent almost four years attenuating just
one strain, or, as it turned out, one type (II).

The existence of three types of polio virus meant
that Cox and Koprowski had to develop not one but
three vaccines. They had to find three strains that
could be safely attenuated and yet remain antigenic,
but they remained confident. It was at that point Koprowski requested permission of the New York State
Department of Health to test the vaccine on some
mentally defective children in a state institution. The
New York officials consulted Rivers. He was vehe-
mently opposed, but Koprowski still got his permission.
It was the report of this test that had so startled and
angered the virologists gathered in Hershey, Pennsylvania, in 1951, as has been mentioned. Koprowski referred to the recipients as "volunteers," but a subsequent reading of his paper on the tests engendered
much speculation about the ability of the subjects to
volunteer for anything. One of the children had to be
fed the chocolate-milk medium through a stomach
tube. There was a great outcry over the ethics of
human experimentation, particularly upon such subjects. Scarcely three years later 400,000 children would
be volunteered by their parents in the greatest feat of
human experimentation ever attempted, and few people seemed concerned about the ethics of it.

No harm came to the mentally defective children
who swallowed the attenuated virus, and all of them
developed antibodies. An interesting observation was
that attenuated virus could be recovered from the feces
of the subjects. This suggested that in the natural

course of things the attenuated virus could be spread to people who did not willfully swallow it. It was recognized that natural, non-paralytic infection was the best way to immunity, and the orally administered vaccine seemed to approach, in concept, a natural, mild infection.

Any joy at this development must have been tempered by the fact that they still had only one attenuated virus, and by the sure knowledge that they had to have three if Lederle was going to have anything to sell in the competitive market. There also existed the possibility that attenuated virus excreted in the stools of vaccinated people could revert to virulence, a possibility that absolutely could not be allowed to happen.

By 1951 Cox and Koprowski certainly knew that polio virus could be grown in tissue culture. Cox, however, had had great success in growing viruses in eggs, and he opted for this method rather than *in vitro* tissue culture. To Cox, the chick embryo in the hen's egg appeared to offer many advantages for virus culture. It was a neat package, prepared by nature, and required none of the elaborate, painstaking procedures of tissue culture. The interior of the egg was sterile to begin with, and the shell protected the egg from contamination. Moreover eggs were cheap, and once a strain had been attenuated by passing it through an animal, it seemed reasonable to suppose that barrels of vaccine virus could be grown with production-line efficiency. Cox also believed that since chickens were never natural hosts of polio virus, an attenuated strain that would grow in chick embryos would never revert to virulence.

The apparent advantages of the chick embryos

were all very encouraging. There was, however, one rather disconcerting disadvantage: polio virus did not grow in them. At least the strains that Cox tried did not grow in the embryos. Cox kept at it, trying one strain after another, perhaps drawing on the reverse inspiration of Sabin and Olitsky, who had given up attempts to grow polio virus in non-nervous tissue after trying only one strain.

After many disappointing failures Cox finally found a strain that would grow in chick embryos. It was the MEF strain, the same one that Salk had used in his vaccine. The MEF strain belonged to Type II, and Cox and Koprowski already had a Type II vaccine. What they really needed was a Type I strain, not to mention a Type III.

While Cox was hopefully injecting one strain after another into hen's eggs, Koprowski was finding more mentally defective children to swallow viruses. Koprowski continued to give the TN strain, and by 1954 he also had a Type I preparation that was a mixture of the Mahoney strain and another, called the Sickle strain. This mixture was called SM, and the children who ingested it remained well and developed antibodies. The SM strain had been attenuated by passing it through mice and cotton rats, but it would not grow in chick embryos. The people at Lederle were still optimistic, but the atmosphere was getting a little edgy. By this time Salk had vaccinated thousands of children in and around Pittsburgh, and the foundation's field trial was in the planning stages. Only the repeated delays of the field trial kept optimism alive that Lederle might still be first.

Even after the Francis report the Lederle team

kept right on going, though with somewhat diminished enthusiasm. The Cutter incident provided renewed motivation for Cox and Koprowski, as the consensus among virologists seemed to swing back to live-virus vaccines.

Sabin started working on attenuating strains in 1953. His early work was not publicized but it no doubt worried Cox and Koprowski. Sabin chose to grow his viruses in the surer medium of tissue culture. Cox still maintained that egg-grown viruses were safer and continued his search for strains adaptable to eggs. Cox, Koprowski, and, no doubt, Sabin could not help being encouraged by the fact that killed-virus vaccine had caused cases of paralytic polio while live vaccines, thus far, had a perfect safety record. They seemed to forget that in preliminary testing Salk's killed-virus vaccine had not caused any polio either. The trouble had been with mass-produced vaccine, and live-virus vaccines had yet to be mass-produced or subjected to mass field trials.

Although Cox and Koprowski had only two attenuated strains they were anxious to carry out larger tests than the limited feedings to institutionalized children. A successful large test would do much to overcome the suspicion and fear engendered among the public and many physicians by the word "live." A demonstration that attenuated strains were safe and effective would also do much to bolster the confidence of Lederle executives, who were beginning to wonder what Cox was hoping to accomplish with all those eggs.

Chances for arranging a large-scale test in the

United States were slim. The Salk-vaccine program had recovered from the Cutter incident and was slowly regaining momentum. The widespread use of Salk vaccine had effectively raised the polio antibody level of millions of children, and there were few, if any, localities with unvaccinated children in sufficient quantities to provide a sample large enough for a valid test of any other vaccine.

Koprowski was frustrated in his efforts to organize trials elsewhere until 1956, when an offer came from a country that has always had more than its share of troubles and continues with that dubious distinction. Dr. George Dick of Queens University in Belfast, Northern Ireland, wrote him to suggest a limited field trial there. For Koprowski it was almost too good to be true. Northern Ireland was a western country, civilized enough to have toilets, sewers, and waterworks. Salk vaccine had not been widely used there, and the general polio antibody level was likely to be low. There were adequate laboratory facilities, a governmental organization that could help to keep track of the subjects, and less bureaucratic red tape than elsewhere.

In most countries of the world, unlike the United States, governmental approval and supervision were required to dose large segments of the population with untried medical products. Koprowski had been unsuccessful in his attempts to induce the British government to approve field trials either in the home island or possessions; but Northern Ireland was largely autonomous as the result of compromises in the treaties with Irish republicans following the rebellions of the 1920s. The various cabinet ministers of Northern Ireland were agreeable to the field trial, and a nod of their heads was sufficient to launch the program without bureaucratic bluster and fuss.

The trials began in 1956 and were very carefully carried out, with more than adequate controls. They were a model of clinical testing, with separate tests being conducted for each of the two strains. The virus was given in a sweet syrup. The volunteers did not get polio and showed a significant rise in antibodies, but they excreted large amounts of virus in their stool, and much of the virus had reverted to virulence in its sojourn through the intestine. The excreted Type II TN strain appeared to be less virulent than the Type I SM, but samples of both types caused paralysis when injected into the brains of monkeys.

In his report Dick recommended that both strains not be used on a large scale. Lederle has never made public the minutes of the frantic board meetings that certainly followed the Belfast trial. The trial and the strains had been largely Koprowski's show, and he left Lederle to become director of the Wistar Institute in Philadelphia. He made it known that he would continue work on attenuated strains.

Usually, in a corporate situation, a man who is in any way responsible for losing several millions of the company's dollars with little hope of recovery is told to start cleaning his desk. Cox not only stayed on at Lederle, but the company demonstrated its confidence in him by continuing to support his search for a live-virus vaccine.

Now there were three separate live-vaccine efforts. Sabin had the support of the National Foundation for

Infantile Paralysis; Cox still had Lederle; Koprowski had only knowledge and enthusiasm and a fraction of the money resources behind Sabin and Cox.

Sabin, an old hand at tissue culture, had chosen to propagate viruses with the proven method of monkey kidney-tissue cultures and had been working on attenuated vaccines since shortly after Salk received the grant to work on the killed-virus vaccine. That Sabin adopted kidney-tissue culture was somewhat ironic, for he and Olitsky, in 1935, had established the tenet of orthodox virology that polio virus would grow only in nerve-tissue culture. That work, and more that followed, established him as one of the more important virologists in the country. By 1948, when Enders was growing polio virus in non-nervous tissue, Sabin had accomplished much in a brilliant career, and the revelation that he had made a mistake in 1935 did not make the slightest dent in his reputation.

As a young man Sabin had to fight harder and longer than any of the other principals on the polio scene to achieve his goals. He was born in 1906 in Bialystok, a city which was then in Russia but is now in Poland. Bialystok had a reputation for the poverty of its inhabitants, and the Sabin family fitted the pattern. He and his parents came to the United States in 1921, and young Sabin lived with relatives in Paterson, New Jersey, where he went to high school. An uncle offered to pay his college tuition on condition that Sabin go to dental school. He accepted and actually went to dental school for two years. Years later, in an interview with a *Time* reporter, Sabin said that reading Paul de Kruif's

Microbe Hunters had inspired him to leave dental school, forsake his uncle's money, and work his way through medical school at New York University.

Sabin, like Salk, spurned a medical practice and chose to do research. At New York University he worked with Dr. William H. Park, the man who had been Brodie's mentor. Early in his career he showed that a skin test for polio, widely in use at the time, was invalid. He was invited to work at the Rockefeller Institute in 1935, only four years after he graduated from medical school. He contributed much to identifying polio as primarily an intestinal disease, which may have helped to convince him of the feasibility of oral vaccine. In 1939 he went to Children's Hospital in Cincinnati.

During the 1954–55 frenzy over the Salk vaccine, Sabin busied himself with verbal broadsides against Salk and quietly went about his own vaccine work. Sabin's over-all strategy was to look for and isolate mutant strains of virus that were non-virulent but still antigenic. He started his search using the laborious technique of diluting suspensions of virus again and again, in an attempt to get as few virus particles as possible in a given suspension. These few particles were then cultured and tested for the desired characteristics. He was not getting any results.

Rivers, who was instrumental in getting foundation support for Sabin's work even at the height of the Salk push, urged Sabin to adopt techniques developed by Renato Dulbecco, a virologist working at the California Institute of Technology. Dulbecco had devised a method of preparing tissue cultures of monkey kidney cells in microscopically thin layers. Diluted virus suspensions were then spread evenly over the culture. Individual colonies of virus, derived from a single virus originally introduced into the culture, could be detected by holes—called "plaques"—in the cell layer, caused by the activity of the virus. The virus could then be isolated, recultured, and tested to determine if it was a mutant with the desired characteristics of non-virulence and antigenicity.

With this technique Sabin made rapid progress. In the course of his work he tried his strains on 10,000 monkeys and 160 chimpanzees. In 1956 he felt that he was ready for testing. Following tradition, the first experimental human feedings were given to himself and his family. He followed with feedings to some 200 inmates of federal penitentiaries. Neither he nor his family nor the convicts got polio, and all of them showed raised antibody levels for all three types. Sabin also had to look around for a suitable place to hold a mass field trial. The United States was out of the question for the same reasons it had been for Cox and Koprowski. When Sabin announced that he was going to hold field trials in the Soviet Union there was initial surprise. On closer examination it was clear that Sabin had made a brilliant move.

The USSR had only recently begun to have a polio problem, and amenities had improved to the point where children were not likely to have high antibody levels. There were many other advantages. The nature of the Soviet government guaranteed that there would be complete control over all aspects of the field trial. Once the rulers of the country agreed to the trial, everything that had to be done would be done without hindrance from dissenters. A persistent news corps, which had so plagued Salk, would not exist. The situation in the USSR was in marked contrast to the United States, where the media provided a blow-by-blow account of all events from polio shots to space shots.

Sabin sent samples of his three strains of attenuated mutant virus to the Russian virologist Anatoli Smorodintsev. Smorodintsev and another virologist, Mikhel P. Chumakov, were in charge of the field-trial operations. They tested the strains for virulence and found mild reactions in monkeys after injection of virus into the spinal cord. The Russians nevertheless went ahead with the field trial with full confidence that eating virus suspended in syrup or candy was one thing and having it injected directly into one's spinal cord was quite another. Distribution of the vaccine started in the spring of 1957, and in typical Russian fashion nothing more was heard about the progress of the trial until a formal report was made in 1959.

Meanwhile there was ample media coverage of the 1957–59 activities of Cox and Koprowski. In late 1957 Koprowski carried out a limited test in the former Belgian Congo. (The Belgian colonial administration had improved sanitation to the point where polio was beginning to be a minor problem.) Koprowski had attenuated strains only for Types I and III, which he fed in a sweet syrup; some 240,000 individuals were involved, and there was even a small epidemic, which started unexpectedly as the trials began. The epidemic did wane as the trials proceeded, but there was no way of knowing if the vaccine had been responsible for ending the epidemic. No harm came to the volunteers, but follow-up studies were almost impossible. Laboratory facilities were inadequate, and the subjects had a habit of disappearing before blood and stool samples could be taken. A curious thing about this trial was that Koprowski apparently claimed that the World Health Organization had supported him, while the organization denied that it had helped him in any way.

Cox was working in Nicaragua, Uruguay, and Colombia. He had the support of the Pan-American Health Organization. In March of 1958 there was an epidemic in Colombia. Salk vaccine was shipped in but could not be used effectively in an epidemic situation. Too much time was required between shots, and it was very difficult to get people to come back for second and third shots. Colombian officials asked for Lederle vaccine. As in the Congo, the epidemic subsided but it was impossible to determine if it was due to the live vaccine.

For types I and II Cox used his SM and the MEF strains, respectively. The type III strain was called "Fox," after Dr. John Fox of Tulane University, who extracted it from a one-year-old child with non-paralytic polio. Cox fed all three strains at once, suspended in a syrup, while Koprowski and Sabin fed them separately. Cox felt that his method was convenient, but Sabin and Koprowski thought that the strains might interfere with one another. The interference factor was later shown to be negligible, and today all three strains are usually taken together.

It became known that the results of the first phase

of the Sabin field trial in Russia would be revealed at the International Conference on Live-Virus Vaccines to be held in Washington in June 1959. The meeting was planned by the World Health Organization and the Pan-American Health Organization. All three contenders were to present papers, but Sabin's report was considered to be the main event. That the results of the trial were favorable was obvious when the Russians announced that they were coming to the meeting. They would not have made an appearance if the trial had been unsuccessful. The only question was, just how successful.

In addition to Russia and some of the satellite countries, Sabin vaccine had also been dispensed in Mexico and, during a 1958 epidemic, in Singapore. The Singapore trial was interesting in that Sabin employed a tactic that ensured his vaccine would get the credit for stopping the epidemic. The Singapore epidemic was primarily a Type I outbreak. However, Type II vaccine was fed on the theory that infection by one type tended to interfere with infection by another. Among the vaccinated there were no Type II cases and six Type I cases, a result far more impressive than Cox and Koprowski had managed in Colombia and the Congo respectively.

The Singapore results, published in the *British Medical Journal* in early 1959, had increased the excitement surrounding the Washington meeting—and what Sabin read at the meeting was nothing short of spectacular. The numbers alone were overpowering: 4,500,000 people in the USSR, Poland, Czechoslovakia, Singapore, and Mexico had taken the vaccine. The size

of the sample made Salk's field trial of 400,000 partici-
pants seem insignificant. There were no ill effects and
the increase in antibodies was impressive. All that had
been heard before. What the delegates wanted to hear
was information on reversion to virulence.

Perhaps the greatest fear about live vaccines was
that attenuated viruses might revert to virulence, as indeed had been the case in the Belfast trials. Again, the
Russian results were spectacular. Smorodintsev reported that he had repassed attenuated virus through
the intestines of children as many as eight times; in
monkeys, there had been a slight increase in virulence
after direct injection of virus into the spinal cord.

Sabin and the Russians put on a good show, made
even better by the admission of the slight increase in
virulence. There was a mistrust of Russians brought on
by ten years of "cold war," and if the report had been
100 per cent favorable, concealment and even falsifica-
tion of information might have been suspected. Almost
everyone in attendance was enormously impressed.
Cox and Koprowski delivered reports, but hardly anyone bothered to listen.

There followed a series of international meetings
through the rest of 1959 and into 1960. Sabin strength-
ened his position, while Cox made futile attempts to
chase and overtake him. Sabin so overwhelmed the virology world that at the Sixth European Symposium on
Poliomyelitis, held in Munich in September 1959, Cox
was not even invited to speak. The excuse was offered
that Cox, as a representative of industry, could not appear at a "meeting of scientists." After much corporate

bellowing and stamping, a substitute, Dr. Henry Bauer, director of the Minnesota Public Health Laboratories, was allowed to present the Lederle view.

At each succeeding meeting Sabin's achievement came across as more impressive. At Munich he reported that 6,000,000 persons had been vaccinated and that virus had been recovered and passed through the intestines of children as many as ten times with negligible reversion to virulence. A month later, at a meeting of the United States Public Health Service, the number of the vaccinated had increased to 10,000,000. At the Fifth International Poliomyelitis Conference in July 1960 the number was reported as approaching 15,-000,000.

Nevertheless there was still some apprehension over reversion to virulence. The officials at the National Institutes of Health were not going to allow themselves to be rushed into licensing, as had been the case with the Salk vaccine. The pressure for live vaccine, however, was increasing, and it was conceded that one live-virus vaccine or another would eventually be licensed. It only remained to make the choice between Cox's and Sabin's. Koprowski was no longer in the running. He had nothing to show. The Belgian Congo had become the Republic of the Congo, and the chaos that followed made the necessary follow-up studies of his trial impossible.

Cox and Sabin now agreed to withhold their mutual accusations and to submit their strains to testing by an independent investigator. The person chosen for this was Joseph Melnick, a virologist in Houston, Texas. His work was widely referred to as the "Melnick arbitration." When Melnick was done, he was not too happy with either Cox's or Sabin's strains, but he was far unhappier with Cox's, which proved to be much more virulent.

Cox was not ready to surrender, and in 1960 he had two more opportunities to test. The first occurred because of dissatisfaction with the results from Salk vaccine in Dade County, Florida, which contains Miami. Among about fifty cases of paralytic polio, there were seven who had received the full regimen of three Salk vaccine injections. Two of these cases died. Dade County was ready to try a live-virus vaccine, and the Cox-Lederle vaccine was the choice. Even though there was no official indication that Dade County chose Lederle because the Sabin vaccine was "tainted" by association with the Soviets, this may indeed have been a factor in the decision, a suspicion increased by the fact that 1960 was an election year.

The second opportunity was an offshoot of "cold war" diplomacy. The international political situation had kept the Sabin vaccine out of West Berlin while it had been widely dispensed in East Germany and the other satellite nations. An epidemic in West Berlin would have been extremely embarrassing to the Western powers. Sabin's "Russian" vaccine was out of the question in West Berlin, so Lederle was requested to supply the vaccine. This was done in May 1960, and some 280,000 children were vaccinated.

The Fifth International Poliomeylitis Conference convened in Copenhagen on July 26, 1960. It was too soon to know the results of the Miami and West Berlin vaccinations; but according to rumors spread in the bars, restaurants, and hotel-room receptions, the Cox programs were in trouble.

The intrigues, maneuvering, and politicking were more obvious than they had been at previous conferences. The atmosphere was worse than that at the 1954 conference. It was like a trade show. Supporters of Cox and Sabin acted like salesmen, collaring delegates in corners, wining and dining people who were supposed to be important. There were even free samples. Confident Russians strolled through the hotel lobbies handing out pieces of candy containing live attenuated virus.

There were also Salk supporters at the conference, along with Salk himself. His presence was almost embarrassing. Those seeking favor from Sabin, the apparent winner, were afraid to be seen near Salk. Salk's cause was not helped by reports of the polio situation in the United States in 1959. The number of cases, although well below the peak year of 1952, was double the 1957 level. An epidemic in Massachusetts was particularly disturbing, since the Salk-vaccine program in that state had been well run and many had received three shots.

In his talk Salk maintained that the upsurge in cases in 1959 was due, not to ineffectiveness of his vaccine, but to failure to take it. Such statements seemed to strengthen the contention of Sabin supporters that the main shortcoming of the Salk vaccine was that it was nearly impossible to get everyone to take the full course of three or four shots.

The full results of the Miami and West Berlin programs were revealed after the conference, and the only interpretation that could be made was disaster for Cox. There were cases of paralytic polio among the vaccinated in both Florida and Germany. Although it was never conclusively proved that Lederle vaccine caused the paralysis, the rub was that there *were* cases in Lederle-vaccinated children and none had occurred during the Sabin trial. There no longer seemed to be any choice. On August 24, 1960, Surgeon-General Leroy Burney announced that his office would recommend the licensing of the Sabin vaccine. He stated, however, that he would proceed cautiously and that the Public Health Service had been instructed to form a special Oral Poliomyelitis Vaccine Advisory Committee to make final judgments. There was nothing for Lederle to do but salvage what they could from the situation. On the same day as the Surgeon-General's announcement, Lederle made it known that it had contracted to manufacture Sabin vaccine.

There were still some official trepidations about the Sabin vaccine, primarily because there was no way of knowing if the Russians had concealed any instances of vaccine-induced paralysis. However, some 15,-000,000 Eastern Europeans had received the vaccine with no indication of large numbers of cases of paralytic polio. That would have been difficult to conceal even in Russia.

This time the church bells did not ring. No *Thank you, Dr. Sabin* signs went up in store windows. No proposals were made for Sabin dimes. There was no presidential citation or any of the rest of the canonizing syndrome that had greeted Salk. The people had grown weary of polio heroes.

Sabin did receive one accolade that was completely unprecedented. On June 28, 1961, the House of Delegates of the AMA Convention voted approval of the Sabin vaccine. This had not been done for the Salk vaccine, nor had it ever been done for any other medical product. There was no televised report, but a drug company, Charles Pfizer, one of the largest manufacturers of the Sabin vaccine, did show a company-made film.

There followed the predictable demand for Sabin vaccine. Again, there were long lines of children in school gymnasiums, armories, and public auditoriums. This time they lined up, not with rolled-up sleeves, but with mouths open to receive sugar cubes moistened with live-virus suspension, or live virus in spoonfuls of syrup. There was at least one known case of involuntary vaccine-swallowing. A man answering an ad for an assistant custodian's job walked into the gymnasium of a Connecticut school while hundreds of noisy students were milling about waiting for vaccine. Since the school nurse looked like someone official, he approached her to ask where he could find the chief custodian, and as he opened his mouth to speak the harried nurse popped a sugar cube into it.

The Sabin vaccine was licensed on a strain-by-strain basis. Type I was released in August 1961, Type II in October 1961. Type III was not licensed until March 1962. (The Salk vaccine continued in licensed status.) By the time the Type I strain was licensed, Sabin and his Russian colleagues claimed that 77,-000,000 people had received the vaccine without ill effect. The relative ease of manufacture, compared to the Salk vaccine, and the months of deliberation before licensing seemed to insure that there would be no mishaps such as the Cutter incident. But Sabin would soon be painfully reminded that the big vats of the drug companies were not the same as the test tubes and Petri dishes in the research laboratory.

The companies had had some difficulty with the Type III virus, which sometimes showed a tendency to revert to virulence. The offered explanations of "production problems" were ominously reminiscent of similar statements in 1953 and 1954. Joseph Melnick had had nothing good to say about Sabin's Type III strain during his arbitration tests. He had observed that some Type III virus that had passed through human intestine caused paralysis when injected into the spinal cords of monkeys. The Advisory Committee of the Public Health Service had been worried about this but eventually conceded that the vaccine was, after all, eaten and not injected into human spinal cords. And 77,000,000 vaccinated Eastern Europeans seemed proof of the vaccine's safety.

The first reports of paralysis among vaccinated people began to come in around July 1962. Predictably, the first reaction was that the cases were coincidental. But the Cutter specter reappeared as it became known that almost all the cases were caused by Type III, that they had occurred approximately thirty days after ingestion of the vaccine, and that the victims had not received Salk vaccine. By the beginning of September there were some sixty known vaccine-associated cases, almost all of whom were adults.

The picture of a haggard Sabin that appeared in

Life magazine was almost a copy of the picture of a haggard Salk that had appeared in the same magazine eight years before, during the Cutter crisis. There was no way to obtain positive proof that the vaccine had caused the cases, but the circumstantial evidence was very strong. Again there were urgent investigations as the Advisory Committee met to consider the problem. Dr. Luther L. Terry, President Kennedy's Surgeon-General, did not follow Scheele's example and stop the Sabin program. He did, however, suggest that Type III vaccine be given only to pre-school and school-age children and to adults only in areas where there were Type III epidemics. The programs for Types I and II continued.

The Advisory Committee investigated the cases and determined that only eleven were "compatible"— that is, definitely associated with the vaccine. There were also a few Type I cases, and four of these were officially designated as "compatible." The Advisory Committee then issued a statement that if the vaccine was to be used for adults it should be "with the full recognition of very small risk." Cries of "Whitewash!" issued from Salk partisans, who maintained that the real number of cases was closer to two hundred.

By the end of 1963 the official figures showed that only eighteen "compatible" cases of paralytic polio occurred among the 70,000,000 Americans who had swallowed the full course of three strains. Again, as in the Salk program, the statistics looked good.

In September 1964 the Public Health Service lowered the "recognition of small risk" age to eighteen. It advised that persons over eighteen should take the Sabin vaccine only in extraordinary circumstances, such as entering the military service, travel abroad, or in epidemic situations. This advice applied to all the vaccine, not just Type III. The pharmaceutical firms continued to advertise the vaccine in the slick magazines and even in newspapers.

The full cause of the vaccine problems has never been determined. Manufacturing protocols were revised to specify that magnesium chloride be added to the vaccine preparations, and that they be frozen for long-term storage or refrigerated for shorter periods before use. These procedures seem to retard the activity of the virus, and into the 1970s reversion to virulence has not been a problem.

The effort to eliminate polio seemed to have turned full circle. Natural infection has long been recognized as the best road to immunization. In the twentieth century the amenities of civilization have prevented exposure to virus during infancy when such exposure would cause immunity rather than paralysis. No one would dare to propose slipping infants a little dirty food now and then, but children have opened their mouths to receive some sugar "dirtied" with live polio virus. Today most doctors recommend oral polio vaccine in the first year of life, but few stop to think of it as "dirty food."

In 1963 most of the few reported cases of paralytic polio were caused by vaccine virus rather than "wild" virus. In 1964 there were about 110 cases. From 1965 on, paralytic polio has dwindled to virtual non-existence. To the new generation born after the 1960s, poliomyelitis has become what it was to their great-grandfathers at the beginning of the century, an interesting word one might find in a medical dictionary.

EPILOGUE

THE STATUS OF POLIO AS THE RARE DIS-
ease it has become can be maintained only by continuing vaccination programs. That the polio virus still
exists is evident in the small epidemics that occasion-
ally break out in so-called underdeveloped countries,
as these nations acquire the amenities of the machine
age.

Along with the "wild" virus that has always
existed, there now exists, hopefully, "domesticated"
virus, which has been excreted by hundreds of millions
of individuals who have swallowed oral vaccines. The
promoters of live-virus vaccines have always claimed
that this natural spread of excreted virus induces immunity even in those who do not willingly ingest vaccine. Pharmaceutical technology has largely eliminated

the possibility that virus in a vaccine vial will revert to virulence before it is swallowed. However, once this virus passes through the intestine of the original swallower and out into the wide world, no hand of man can change the possibility, indeed probability, that some of this virus might revert to virulence. If such virus re-enters the intestine of an immunized individual, there is no problem. If such virus is introduced into an area inhabited by unvaccinated, non-immune individuals, the result might be disastrous. Such an area could be in an emerging country or in a neglected slum of an American city. There was fear of such an outbreak in the United States in the summer of 1971, and there were campaigns to get vaccine into the mouths of the unvaccinated.

There can be little doubt that since the mid-1960s polio has been submerged by the Sabin vaccine, if only because the Salk vaccine is seldom used anymore. Salk partisans continue to maintain that the number of Sabin-vaccine-induced cases of paralytic polio would have been much higher had the early oral vaccine swallowers in the United States not been protected by Salk vaccine. They also maintain that, given time, the Salk killed-virus vaccine would have virtually eliminated paralytic polio as the Sabin vaccine seems to have done.

That question and many others relative to the vaccines are unanswered; many can never be answered. Just how long immunity induced by Salk vaccine would have lasted will probably never be known, since almost all individuals who received Salk shots subsequently ingested Sabin vaccine. The continuing arguments over which vaccine is better can never be resolved. The most obvious advantage of the Sabin vaccine is that it is swallowed rather than injected. The desire to avoid pain is strong, and the necessity of returning for second and third shots has definitely been a deterrent.

The Salk vaccine was far from perfect. The cases dropped sharply from 1954 on, but there were some 2000 reported cases in 1959. People died from receiving improperly prepared vaccine, though the Cutter incident was not the first time people died from badly prepared or improperly administered medications, nor was it the last. The Cutter incident was part of the price paid for the frantic rush into a vaccine program, after some thirty years of delay and inaction brought about by misleading information on the nature of the polio virus. Whatever shortcomings the Salk vaccine may have had, they have been overshadowed by the thousands of people who have remained alive and unparalyzed, who might not have been so had they not taken Salk shots.

A great price was paid for the vaccines of the 1950s and 1960s, and the money involved was the least of it. Scientific endeavor was frequently reduced to the level of merchandising, and the alleged objectivity of scientists was severely strained in the intensity of competition. It was a vivid reminder that science had become big business with all its attendant problems.

The commercialization of science started long before the polio-vaccine spectacle. Ever since governments and all varieties of entrepreneurs realized that useful products could result from the application of observed phenomena explained by scientists, pressure has been exerted on scientists to spend more time on designing things and less time building theories.

Shortly after the Salk-vaccine field trial, the National Foundation for Infantile Paralysis was convinced that polio was no longer a problem and accordingly dropped "for Infantile Paralysis" from its name and became simply the National Foundation-March of Dimes. It has remained an active organization, with Basil O'Connor serving as its president until his death in March 1972. The foundation's activities have been directed toward raising money for research in birth defects and various genetically transmitted diseases. Jonas Salk has continued to benefit from foundation largesse as the director of the Salk Institute for Biological Studies in La Jolla, California, which was set up with foundation funds in 1960.

The successful fund-raising efforts of the National Foundation have encouraged the formation of other organizations dedicated to the "conquest" of various diseases, such as muscular dystrophy, cystic fibrosis, and multiple sclerosis. These are relatively rare afflictions, and far more prevalent diseases, particularly sickle-cell anemia, have not attracted the attention of private fund-raising organizations. Muscular dystrophy and cystic fibrosis are genetically transmitted diseases, which primarily affect white children. Sickle-cell anemia is also genetically transmitted but is found exclusively in black populations. Only in recent years has sickle-cell anemia attracted the interest of governmental health agencies.

In its time the campaign against polio attracted more public interest and gathered greater totals of voluntary small donations than any other medical research. The efforts of the muscular dystrophy and cystic fibrosis groups are feeble by comparison, even with their occasional twenty-four-hour "telethons," during which big-name entertainers direct broadsides at television viewers in hopes of turning them into big givers.

While muscular dystrophy and cystic fibrosis are relatively rare diseases, the malignant diseases, collectively called cancer, are not. In the wake of President Nixon's declaration of a "cancer crusade" in 1971, there will occur the greatest public participation in medical research in the history of the world. Every American taxpayer will be a participant, willingly or not.

The cancer crusade is the culmination of the trend toward increased government participation in medical research in the years following World War II. To many Americans so massive a commitment to a health program was refreshing news after so many years of a tragic war in Southeast Asia and violent protest at home. It seemed a first step in the much called for realignment of priorities for domestic needs. To much of the scientific community, however, the presidential announcement was cause for alarm—not by the prospect of more national resources allocated for medical research, but by the effect of increased public and congressional attention on the nature of the research.

As the years pass and thousands of millions of dollars are poured into cancer research with no "cure" in sight, some congressmen will surely call for investigations into "waste and duplication." Such investigations into research supported by the National Institutes of Health did indeed occur in the 1960s. Political pressure could result in the allocation of more funds for the spectacular kind of research that impresses congress-men rather than for more prosaic research the value of which is understood only by scientists—such as the work of Enders, who in his own quiet way developed a vaccine for measles in 1963, with the collaboration of Thomas Peebles, a Boston pediatrician.

The National Foundation employed such phrases as "significant breakthrough" and "encouraging devel-opment" to stimulate the public into a giving mood; those concerned with cancer research might be forced to use similar tactics to stimulate congressmen into an appropriating mood. There remains the specter raised by President Johnson in 1966 when he wanted to know "if too much energy was being spent on basic re-search and not enough on translating laboratory find-ings into tangible benefits for the American people." This was indicative of the general lack of knowledge that "energy spent on basic research" has always been a necessary prerequisite to "tangible benefits."

A national cancer-research program, funded by congressional appropriations, could be subject to the same pressures that forced the shoddy, deadly Brodie vaccine into the arms of children in 1935, and forced the Salk vaccine into use after only a two-hour deliber-ation. The same sort of problems could arise with re-spect to leukemia. If specific types of viruses are defi-nitely linked to some forms of leukemia—and there is a growing body of evidence that this may be so—then the possibility of a vaccine, albeit remote at this point, cannot be overlooked. Since many forms of leukemia are prevalent in children there is, as there was with polio, a great deal of emotion associated with this affliction. "Breakthroughs" in leukemia-virus research could result in pressures from Congress and the public to make a leukemia vaccine before there is enough basic information on the virus-host relationship and before the problems of mass production are sufficiently investigated. There could again be canonization of vaccine heroes, and the furious triumphs and tragedies of the polio vaccine in the first half of this century could well be repeated in the second half. Only the name of the disease will be changed.

GLOSSARY
CHRONOLOGY
BIBLIOGRAPHY
INDEX

GLOSSARY

ADJUVANT.   A substance injected with a drug or a vaccine that releases the vaccine gradually from the injection site and enhances and prolongs the action of the vaccine.

ANTIBODY.   A protein substance in blood that fights off infection by combining with the disease-causing substance and neutralizing it.

ANTIGEN.   A substance that stimulates the body to produce antibodies.

ATTENUATION.   The process of weakening disease organisms by passage through animals or cell cultures.

BACTERIOLOGY.   The science that deals with the study of bacteria.

BACTERIOPHAGE.   A virus that invades bacterial cells and reproduces within them.

BULBAR POLIOMYELITIS.   Invasion of nerve cells in the medulla oblongata, the lowest part of the brain, by polio virus.

CC.   Abbreviation for cubic centimeter, a measure of volume.

CELL.   The basic unit of structure and function in living things.

CELL AND TISSUE CULTURE.   Techniques for growing excised living cells in test tubes and other laboratory glassware.

DNA.   Abbreviation for deoxyribonucleic acid, the hereditary material, or gene.

EMBRYO.   An organism in an early developmental stage.

ENCEPHALITIS.   An inflammation of the brain, usually due to infection by any of several viruses.

ENCEPHALOMYELITIS.   An inflammation of the brain and spinal cord, usually due to infection by any of several viruses.

EPIDEMIOLOGY.   The study of the nature, transmission, and spread of diseases.

GLOBULINS.   Blood proteins that contain antibodies.

HOST.   When an organism is invaded or infected by another organism, the infected individual is called the host.

IMMUNITY.   The state of having sufficient specific antibodies to avoid infection by a specific disease-causing substance.

IMMUNOLOGY.   The study of the nature of immunity.

INFECTIOUS DISEASE.   A disease caused by organisms such as bacteria and viruses.

IN VITRO.   Literally, "in glass"; refers to procedures carried out in laboratory "glassware" (which can be plastic or any number of other materials) rather than in living things (*in vivo*, from the Latin word for "life"). Cell and tissue culture is an example of an *in vitro* procedure.

LEUKEMIA.   A group of blood cancers characterized by an overabundance of white blood cells (leucocytes).

MUTATION.   A change in genes (DNA) that is passed on to succeeding generations.

NEUROLOGY.   The study of the nervous system.

NEUROTROPISM.   A tendency to be attracted to nerve cells. (The adjective is "neurotropic.")

ORGANISM.   A whole living thing.

PANDEMIC.   A widespread, frequently world-wide, outbreak of an infectious disease.

PATHOLOGY.   The study of the effects of disease on cells and tissues.

PLACEBO.   A substance that is dispensed as a medication but is not really a medication.

PLASMA.   The liquid part of the blood; everything except the red blood cells.

PLAQUE.   A hole or patch in a culture of bacteria or viruses that is indicative of the active growth of these organisms.

PNEUMOCOCCUS.   The spherically shaped bacteria that causes pneumonia.

RICKETTSIA.   Microorganisms that are considered intermediate between bacteria and viruses. They are larger than viruses and, like viruses, can multiply only in a living cell.

RNA.   Abbreviation for ribonucleic acid, the nucleic acid that carries the genetic "instructions" from DNA in the nucleus to the rest of the cell.

SERUM.   The liquid part of the blood minus the factors that cause blood-clotting.

STRAIN.   When applied to viruses, strain refers to descendants of a virus that differ in certain respects such as virulence, but do not differ enough to make the descendants a different type.

TMV.   Abbreviation for tobacco mosaic virus.

TYPE.   When used in reference to viruses, type refers to viruses that share a similar immunological reaction.

VACCINE.   A substance made of killed disease organisms or modified live disease organisms that, when introduced into the body, stimulates the body to produce antibodies against the particular disease.

VIREMIA.   The presence of virus particles in the blood.

VIROLOGY.   The study of viruses.

VIRULENCE.   The ability of a microorganism to cause disease.

CHRONOLOGY

1796	Jenner uses cowpox pustules to immunize against smallpox.
1885	Pasteur develops attenuated-virus rabies vaccine.
1892–98	Iwanowski (1892) and Beijerinck (1898) describe a filterable agent that causes tobacco mosaic disease.
1908	Landsteiner identifies a virus as cause of poliomyelitis.
1916	First large polio epidemic in the United States.
1931	Elford isolates virus particles with filters.
1935	Stanley isolates and crystallizes TMV virus.
1935	Brodie and Kolmer polio-vaccine disasters.
1935–36	Sabin and Olitsky report that polio virus can be grown only in nerve-tissue cultures.
1936	Theiler develops yellow-fever vaccine.
1942	Virus Research Center set up at Johns Hopkins with funds granted by the National Foundation for Infantile Paralysis.

164

1943	Successful trial of killed-virus influenza vaccine developed by Francis, assisted by Salk.
1944–47	Studies by Bodian, Howe, and Morgan show the existence of three types of polio virus.
1946	Lederle begins live-virus polio vaccine project with Cox and Koprowski. Paul indicated relationship between low standard of living and high level of polio antibodies.
1948	Committee set up by National Foundation for Infantile Paralysis to type polio virus.
1949	Enders, Weller, and Robbins report the culture of polio virus in non-nervous tissue.
1950	Cox and Koprowski swallow their attenuated-polio virus with no ill effect. Morgan and Howe raise polio antibody levels in monkeys through injection of inactivated-virus preparation.
1951	Gamma-globulin field trials. Koprowski reports feeding attenuated live polio virus to mentally defective children.
1952	Bodian and Horstmann demonstrate presence of polio virus in blood of monkeys with pre-paralytic polio. Salk carries out successful tests of inactivated-polio virus preparation at a home for crippled children in Pennsylvania.
1954	Inactivated-virus vaccine field trial (Salk vaccine).
1955	Salk vaccine licensed.
1956	Sabin works on live-virus polio vaccine. Dulbecco's plaqueing techniques used by Sabin. Trial of Lederle vaccine in Belfast, Northern Island.
1957	Initiation of Sabin oral-vaccine field trial in USSR. Koprowski tests his oral vaccine in the Belgian Congo.
1958	Cox tests Lederle oral vaccine in Colombia.
1960	Tests of Lederle vaccine in Dade County, Florida, and West Berlin.
1961–62	Sabin vaccine licensed.
1963	Enders develops measles vaccine.

BIBLIOGRAPHY

Books

Benison, Saul. *Tom Rivers, Reflections on a Life in Medicine and Science.* Cambridge, Mass.: The M.I.T. Press, 1967.

Burnet, F. M., and Stanley, W. M. (eds.). *The Viruses: General Virology.* Vol. 1. New York: Academic Press, 1959.

Carter, Richard, *Breakthrough: The Saga of Jonas Salk.* New York: Trident Press, 1966.

de Kruif, Paul. *Microbe Hunters.* New York: Harcourt, Brace & Co., 1926.

————. *The Fight for Life.* New York: Harcourt, Brace & Co., 1938.

————. *Activities of the National Foundation for Infantile Paralysis in the Field of Virus Research.* New York: National Foundation for Infantile Paralysis, 1939.

Oliver, W. S. *The Man Who Lived for Tomorrow: A Biography of Dr. William H. Park.* New York: E. P. Dutton & Co., 1941.

Paul, J. R. *Clinical Epidemiology.* Chicago: University of Chicago Press, 1958.

———. *A History of Poliomyelitis*. New Haven: Yale University Press, 1971.

Rivers, T. M. *Viral and Rickettsial Infections of Man*. Philadelphia: J. B. Lippincott, 1952.

Schaffer, M., and Muckenfuss, R. S. *Experimental Poliomyelitis*. New York: National Foundation for Infantile Paralysis, 1940.

Stanley, W. M., and Valens, E. G. *Viruses and the Nature of Life*. New York: E. P. Dutton & Co., 1961.

Williams, Greer. *Virus Hunters*. New York: Alfred Knopf, 1959.

Periodicals

Dulbecco, R. "Plaques in monolayer tissue cultures by single particles of an animal virus," *Proceedings of the National Academy of Science*, 38:747 (1952).

Enders, J. F., Weller, T. H., and Robbins, F. C. "Cultivation of the Lansing strain of poliomyelitis virus in cultures of various human embryonic tissues," *Science*, January 28, 1949.

Farrell, L. N., Wood, W., Macmorine, H. G., and Rhodes, A. J., "Cultivation of poliomyelitis viruses in tissue culture," *Canadian Journal of Public Health*, 44:273 (1953).

Francis, T., Jr., and Korns, R. F. "Evaluation of 1954 field trial of poliomyelitis vaccine: synopsis of summary report," *American Journal of Medical Science*, 109:85 (1955).

Hammon, W. "Gamma Globulin in Poliomyelitis," *Scientific American*, July 1952.

Melnick, J. A. "New Era in Polio Research," *Scientific American*, November 1955.

"Recognition for Sabin," *Newsweek*, November 24, 1965.

Robinson, L. W. "Now the Sabin Vaccine for Polio," *New York Times Magazine*, September 6, 1959.

Sabin, A. B. "Present status of attenuated live virus poliomyelitis vaccine," *Bulletin of the New York Academy of Medicine*, 33:17 (1957).

Salk, J. E. "Recent Studies on immunization against poliomyelitis," *Pediatrics*, 12:471 (1953).

———. "Vaccines for Poliomyelitis," *Scientific American*, April 1955.

Strickland, S. P. "Integration of Medical Research and Health Policies," *Science*, September 17, 1971.

Van Riper, H. E. "Progress in the control of paralytic poliomyelitis through vaccination," *Canadian Journal of Public Health*, 46:25 (1955).

INDEX

Allegheny College, 27
American Academy of Pediatrics, 99
American Cyanamid Company, Lederle Division, 59-60, 127-29, 132-34, 136-67, 141, 144-45, 147
American Medical Association, 81, 95, 105, 123, 148
American Red Cross, 61
antibodies, 35, 38, 50, 53, 56, 60-61, 63-64, 67, 72-76, 79-80, 99, 130-31, 135, 139, 143
Aureomycin, 128
Avery, Oswald, 26-27

bacteria, 5, 29-31, 34-35, 56, 77, 98, 129; *Escherichia*
coli, 77; pneumococcus, 26-27
bacteriophage(s), 77-78
Bauer, Henry, 144
Beijerninck, Martinus, 28-29
Belgian Congo, Republic of the, trials of oral Koprowski vaccine, 140-44
Bell, Joseph, 89-90, 92, 96
Birthday Ball Committee, 21
Black Plague, 3-4
Bodian, David, 47-48, 50, 63-64, 76, 87, 101, 112, 129
Brebner, William, 51-52
British Medical Journal, 142
Brodie, Maurice, 20-23, 34, 38, 48-49, 71, 78, 100, 116, 124, 129, 138. *See also* poliomyelitis vaccines
Burney, Leroy, 147

California Institute of Technology, 138
California, State of, Department of Public Health, 116
cancer, 156-57
Cantor, Eddie, 17
cell and tissue culture, 35-36, 56-58, 66-67, 69, 72, 80, 114, 125-26, 132, 134, 137-139
Chase, Martha, 77-78
Children's Hospital (Boston), 56
Children's Hospital (Cincinnati), 138
Chloromycetin, 84
cholera, 6
Chumakov, Mikhel, 140
City College of New York, 24
Cohn, Edwin, 60
Colombia, 141, 142; polio epidemic in, 141
Columbia University, 48
Commonwealth Fund, 47
Cox, Herald, 59-60, 93, 127-34, 136, 139-47. *See also* poliomyelitis vaccines
Crick, Francis, 78
Cutter Company, 95, 116-20, 122-23, 125, 134-35, 149-50, 154
cystic fibrosis, 155-56

Dade County, Florida, trials of Cox-Lederle vaccine, 145-47
de Kruif, Paul, 19-20, 100, 137
deoxyribonucleic acid (DNA), 27, 77-78
d'Herelle bodies, 77
d'Herelle, Felix H., 77

Dick, George, 135-36
diphtheria, 4-5, 110
Dulbeco, Renato, 138
Dyer, Robert, 116

Eisenhower, Dwight D., 98, 112-13
Elford, William, 29
encephalitis, 33, 35, 46
Enders, John, 55-59, 61-62, 66, 68, 71, 81, 87-88, 108, 112, 114, 121, 124-25, 127, 129, 137, 157
epidemic(s), 3, 6-7, 9-10, 31, 34, 37, 60, 117, 119, 140-42, 146, 151-52
equine encephalitis, 43

formalin, 71, 73-74, 121
Fox, John, 141
Francis, Thomas, 26-28, 36-41, 43, 48, 50, 68, 71, 89, 96-97, 103-104, 107-12, 117, 123-24, 133

gamma globulin, 60-61, 63, 71, 119; field trials of, 62-63, 70, 76, 94
Gard, Sven, 105, 114
Garroway, Dave, 110
Gebhardt, Louis, 122
Griffith, Fred, 27

Hammon, William, 50, 62, 70, 87, 112, 125
hepatitis, 56, 62
Hershey, A. D., 77-78
Hobby, Oveta Culp, 98, 111-13, 118, 123
Horstmann, Dorothy, 63-64, 85

House Committee on Interstate and Foreign Commerce, hearing on vaccine appropriation, 123-25
Howard Medical School, 56
Howe, Howard, 47-48, 59, 69, 87, 91, 129

immunity, 7-8; induced, 32-33, 99, 109-10, 152; natural, 9, 132, 151; passive, 67-70; to polio virus, 20, 27, 48, 54; to viral diseases, 30-31, 38-39
infantile paralysis, see poliomyelitis
influenza, 7, 27-28; vaccines, 36-40, 43, 48, 89-91
International Conference on Live Virus Vaccines, 142
International Polio Congress (Conference): Fifth, 144-45; Second, 69; Third, 105
International Symposium on Poliomyelitis, Sixth, 143
Iwanowski, Dmitri, 28-29

Jenner, Edward, 31-32, 85
Johns Hopkins School of Public Health and Hygiene, 42-43, 47-48, 55, 63, 125
Johnson, Lyndon B., 157
Journal of the American Medical Association, The, 82

Karolinska Institutet (Stockholm), 114
Kennedy, John F., 150
Kolmer, John, 21-23, 34, 48-49, 78-79, 124, 129. See also poliomyelitis vaccines

Koprowski, Hilary, 59-60, 68-69, 76, 78, 85, 94, 105, 127-37, 139-44. See also poliomyelitis vaccines
Kramer, Sidney, 60

Ladies Home Journal, The, 81
Landsteiner, Karl, 33-34
leukemia, 157-58
Life magazine, 115, 150
Lilly, Eli, Company, 95, 97, 99, 108, 122

McCarty, Maclyn, 26
McGinnes, A. Foard, 95
MacLeod, Colin M., 26
magnesium chloride, 151
March of Dimes (campaign), see National Foundation for Infantile Paralysis
"March of Time, The," 17
Mayer, Manfred, 125
Maxcy, Kenneth, 47
measles vaccine, 157
Melnick, Joseph, 144-45, 149
merthiolate, 98, 106, 111
Michael Reese Hospital, 92-93
Michigan, State of, Department of Health, 60
Michigan, University of, 36-37, 41, 97, 108
Microbe Hunters, 20, 138
Milzer, Albert, 92-93
Minnesota Public Health Laboratories, 144
Morgan, Isabel, 47-48, 59, 61, 69, 129
Morgan, Thomas Hunt, 48
Mount Sinai Hospital, 36, 114
multiple sclerosis, 155
mumps, 56
muscular dystrophy, 155-56

National Academy of Sciences, 114
National Broadcasting Company, 110
National Foundation for Infantile Paralysis, 9, 16, 18-19, 23, 37, 42, 45-47, 51-52, 56, 59-60, 64, 68, 78-79, 82-83, 85, 110, 155, 157; gamma globulin program of, 60-62, 70-71, 76, 94; March of Dimes campaign, 17, 50, 76, 81, 97, 104; Sabin program, 136, 138; Salk program, 70, 75, 79-81, 83-106, 118-19, 121, 123, 128, 133, 138; Salk vaccine trial evaluation, 97, 103, 107-09, 111-13; Vaccine Advisory Committee of, 86, 88, 91-92, 95-96, 100-01, 106; Virus Research Committee, 21-22, 43; Virus Typing Committee (Immunization Committee), 50, 53-54, 62-63, 66-67, 69, 80-81, 87, 91, 101
National Foundation—March of Dimes, 155
National Institute for Medical Research (England), 29
National Institutes of Health, 89, 92, 116, 121-22, 144, 158; contract with National Foundation for testing and licensing of Salk vaccine, 97-99, 101, 106-07, 113; Laboratory of Biologics Control of, 90, 104, 112-13, 123
National Research Council, 37
National Tuberculosis Association, 12-13, 15

New York State Department of Health, 131
New York Times, The, 16, 77
New York University, School of Medicine, 20, 22, 26, 36, 138
Nixon, Richard M., 156
Northern Ireland, trials of Cox-Koprowski vaccine, 135-36, 143
nucleic acid, 77-78

O'Connor, Basil, 14-16, 18, 20-22, 42-47, 51, 61, 67, 69, 71, 81, 83, 85-87, 93-97, 101, 103-04, 106-07, 110, 112, 119, 121, 155
Olitsky, Peter, 35, 48, 58, 132, 137
Oral Poliomyelitis Vaccine Advisory Committee (Public Health Service), 148-50

Pan-American Health Organization, 142; trials of Cox vaccine, 141
pandemic(s), 7, 27, 38
Park, William H., 138
Parke Davis Company, 83-84, 95, 97-99
Pasteur Institute, 77
Pasteur, Louis, 11, 20, 29, 32-33, 59, 85, 128, 130
Paul, John, 50, 64
Peebles, Thomas, 157
Pennsylvania, University of, 48, 56
Pfizer, Charles, Company, 148
Phipps, James, 32
Pittman Moore Company, 95
Pittsburgh, University of, Medical School, 41, 49-50;

Graduate School of Public Health, 70

pneumonia, 26-27

poliomyelitis, 10, 13, 19, 23, 37, 42, 45, 47, 51, 60, 63-64, 79, 85, 88, 91, 94, 152, 156; antibodies, 54, 64, 70, 74-76, 79-80, 86, 99, 135-36, 139, 143; bulbar spinal paralysis, 109; epidemics of, 3-4, 6-7, 9, 117, 119, 140-42, 146, 151-52; induced immunity to, 99, 109-10, 152; natural immunity to, 9, 132, 151; paralytic symptoms of, 8, 14-16, 64, 116, 119, 149-50; passive immunity to, 67-70; skin test for, 138; in the United States, 3, 6, 7; vaccine-induced cases of, 115-16, 118-21, 134, 141, 147, 149-50, 153-54

poliomyelitis vaccines, 35, 44-45, 56, 58-60, 64, 74-78, 88, 94, 127; Brodie, 20-21, 34, 48-49, 78, 100, 116, 124, 129, 157; Cox (Lederle) oral, 136-37, 140-43; Cox-Koprowski (Lederle) oral, 127-28, 130-34, 136, 141-42; Cutter "disaster," 116-20, 122-23, 125, 134-35, 149-50, 154; development of dead-virus types of, 27, 48, 67-71, 74-75, 79, 84, 87, 89, 93, 105, 115, 124-25, 128, 134, 137; development of live, attenuated types of, 71, 78-80, 87, 105, 127, 130-34, 136-37, 140-41, 143, 146; Kolmer, 21, 34, 48-49, 78-79, 124, 129; Ko-prowski, 140-41, 143; Melnick arbitration of Cox and Sabin vaccines, 144-45, 149. *See also* Sabin vaccine, Salk vaccine

poliomyelitis, viruses of, 8, 20-21, 34-35, 38, 43-46, 48-49, 51-55, 57-58, 61, 64, 66-68, 71-77, 79, 81, 85, 93, 100, 105, 113-15, 120, 122, 124-27, 130, 132-33, 136-37, 143, 151; Lansing strain, 57-58; Fox strain, 141; Mahoney strain, 124-25, 133; MEF strain, 72, 133, 141; mutant strains, 138-40; Saukett strain, 72; sickle strain, 133; SM strain, 133, 136, 141; TN strain, 130, 133, 136; Type I, 72-73, 109, 133, 140-41, 150; Type II, 72, 109, 131, 133, 141-42, 148, 150; Type III, 72, 109, 133, 140, 148-50

President's Birthday Balls, 15-16, 18-21

Priest, Percy, 123

Queens University (Northern Ireland), 135

rabies, 29; vaccines, 31-33, 128; virus of, 34, 128, 130

ribonucleic acid (RNA), 17

rickettsiae, 129

Rivers, Thomas M., 21-22, 43, 46-47, 62, 69, 80-81, 86-87, 93, 106, 108, 111, 117, 124, 131, 138

Robbins, Frederick C., 56, 58-59, 114

Rockefeller Hospital, 21

Rockefeller Institute (Rockefeller University), 21-22, 26-28, 35, 48, 51, 138
Rocky Mountain spotted fever vaccine, 129
Roosevelt, Franklin D., 13-17, 42, 108

Sabin, Albert, 22-24, 35, 44, 50-51, 55, 58-59, 69, 71, 76, 81, 87-88, 91-92, 99, 105, 110, 112-13, 117, 123-25, 132, 136-50, 153, 157
Sabin vaccine (oral), 124, 128, 134, 136, 138-42, 144-51, 153; trials of, 139-43, 147; licensing of, 144, 147, 150
Salk Institute for Biological Studies, 155
Salk, Jonas, 22-26, 36-37, 39-41, 49-51, 55, 59, 66-67, 69-74, 75-76, 79-81, 83, 87, 89-90, 93, 95-96, 98-99, 101, 105-106, 110-14, 117, 119, 121, 124-26, 128, 130, 132-35, 137-38, 140, 143, 145-46, 148-50, 153-55, 157
Salk vaccine, 69-76, 79-90, 93-96, 98-102, 104-06, 109-26, 133-35, 137-38, 141, 143-46, 148-50, 153-54, 157; field trials of, 102-104, 106-107, 111, 113, 115, 118, 133, 143, 155; licensing of, 107, 111-13, 119, 123, 126, 144
Scheele, Leonard A., 111-12, 116-18, 121-23, 150
Schultz, Edwin, 34
Science magazine, 58
Scientific American, 77
Shannon, James, 116

Sharpe and Dohme Company, 95
sickle-cell anemia, 155
Singapore, trial of Sabin vaccine, 142
Smadel, Joseph, 81, 87, 112
smallpox vaccine, 31-32, 85
Smith, Alfred E., 14
Smorodintsev, Anatoli, 140, 143
Stokes, Joseph, Jr., 56, 61-62
Stanford University, 34
Stanley, Wendell, 29-30, 124-25

Temple University, 21
Terry, Luther L., 150
Theiler, Max, 81, 85
Theiler's disease, 101
tobacco mosaic disease, 28-29
tuberculosis, 4, 13, 98
Tulane University, 141
Turner, Thomas, 87
typhoid fever, 4-5, 110
typhus vaccine, 129

United Research Council, 37
United States: government participation in disease research, 155-58; laws to protect health, 50
United States Public Health Service, 100, 144, 147, 148-50. See also National Institutes of Health
USSR, field trials of Sabin oral vaccine in, 139-40, 142-43, 145, 147-49
Utah, University of, 122

vaccine(s), 5-6; bacterial, 36, 85; development of dead-virus types, 28, 38-40, 124; development of live-virus types, 31-33, 36-38, 40, 56, 123, 130, 141; distemper, 62; encephalitis, 48; influenza, 36-40, 48, 89-91; measles, 157; mumps, 56; rabies, 31-33, 85, 128; Rocky Mountain spotted fever, 129; smallpox, 85; typhus, 129; yellow fever, 85. *See also* poliomyelitis vaccines

Van Riper, Hart, 91-93, 96, 100

viremia, 76

virus(es), 28-29, 31; bacteriophages, 77; influenza, 36-39; leukemia, 158; mumps, 56-57; Q fever, 129; rabies, 32-33, 128, 130; strains of, 29-39, 48-49, 58, 130, 138; Tobacco Mosaic Virus, 29-30. *See also* poliomyelitis virus

Virus Typing Project, 50-55, 69

Warm Springs, Georgia, 14-16, 20

Warsaw Conservatory of Music, 129

Warsaw Medical School, 129

Watson Home for Crippled Children, Salk vaccine trials, 79-81, 96

Watson, James D., 78

Weaver, Harry, 45-46, 49-50, 66-68, 80, 91-92

Welles, Thomas H., 56, 58-59, 114

West Berlin, Germany, trials of Cox-Lederle vaccine, 145-47

Wilson, Earl, 82-83, 100

Winchell, Walter, 100

Wistar Institute, 136

Workmann, William, 112-13

World Health Organization, 141-42

Wyeth Company, 95

Yale University School of Medicine, 27

yellow fever, 6; vaccines against, 31, 85

Zinsser, Hans, 56

About the Author

Aaron E. Klein was born in Atlanta, Georgia, and received his B.A. in zoology from the University of Pennsylvania in 1953. He received his M.S. from the University of Bridgeport in 1958 and has also studied at Yale University. A former public school and college teacher in the biological sciences, he is currently in educational publishing as managing editor of the science department for a leading publisher. He is the author of *Threads of Life: Genetics from Darwin to DNA* and *The Hidden Contributors: Black Scientists and Inventors in America,* among other books.